Contributors

Gifford Batstone *Consultant Chemical Pathologist, Salisbury General Hospital, Odstock, Salisbury, Wiltshire SP2 8BJ*

David Bowden *Managing Director, Merrett Health Risk Management Ltd, 60 West Street, Brighton, Sussex BN1 2RB*

Bob Broughton *formerly Co-ordinator and Adviser, Medical Audit Wales, Welsh Health Common Services Authority, Heron House, 35–43 Newport Road, Cardiff CF2 1SB; now Welsh Secretary, British Medical Association, 1 Cleeve House, Cardiff Business Park, Llanishen, Cardiff CF4 5GJ*

Kenneth Calman *Chief Medical Officer, Department of Health, Richmond House, 79 Whitehall, London SW1A 2NS*

Peter Coe *District General Manager, East London and The City Health Authority, Tredegar House, 97–99 Bow Road, London E3 2AN*

David Colin-Thome *General Practitioner, The Health Centre, Chester Close, Castlefields, Runcorn, Cheshire WA7 2HY*

Graham Coomber *formerly District General Manager, North Worcestershire District Health Authority, The Croft, Sutton Park Road, Kidderminster, Bromsgrove DY11 6LJ; now Chief Executive, North Birmingham Healthcare Purchasing Consortium, 1 Verna Road, Birmingham B16 9SA*

David Dunn *Consultant Surgeon, Addenbrooke's Hospital, Hills Road, Cambridge CB2 2QQ*

Raymond Godwin *Chairman, Royal College of Radiologists Audit Working Party, X–Ray Department, West Suffolk Hospital, Hardwick Lane, Bury St Edmunds, Suffolk IP33 2QZ*

Anthony Hopkins *Director, Research Unit, Royal College of Physicians of London, 11 St Andrews Place, London NW1 4LE*

Patricia Kent *Regional Audit Co-ordinator, Yorkshire Regional Health Authority, and Chair, Medical Audit Association, The Queen Building, Park Parade, Harrogate HG1 5AH*

Contents

Section 3: INFORMATION MANAGEMENT, INFORMATION TECHNOLOGY AND CLINICAL AUDIT

Section 4: MANAGERS AND CLINICAL AUDIT, AND RESOURCES FOR AUDIT

Section 5: ACHIEVING CHANGE

Introduction: Future directions of audit

Kenneth Calman
Chief Medical Officer, Department of Health

Clinical audit should be seen within the broader framework of quality of service to patients. It is a method for assisting in delivering quality, and as such needs to be related to other initiatives. Quality is about values. The values of individuals, of communities, and of professionals determine what is most important for them. If providing a high quality of care is a value which *is* important, professional staff will wish to use any method, including audit, which will enhance that care. Values also determine priorities and set the tone, or culture, of the clinical service unit.

At the end of the day, it is *outcomes* which are important for the patient or the community. Thus, what matters will be an understanding of what is meant by outcomes and how they are measured. Only by looking at outcomes will it be possible to use resources effectively and improve the quality of care delivered. However, some audit projects are process based, which is entirely proper if these are seen as means to improving the outcome of care.

Some background

Medical audit as an initiative of the Department of Health as part of the National Health Service (NHS) reforms began in 1989, although I acknowledge the work of many individuals before then. Since 1989, over £150 million has been spent in England on the development of the process. Several years into the initiative in 1993, it is a good time to review progress and consider the future. In addition, the National Audit Office has embarked on an investigation of the current position of clinical audit. This adds pressure on us to ensure, first, that there is good 'value for money' in the progress so far and, secondly, that there is a clear vision for the future.

Clinical audit is not a new process, but has been part of professional practice for generations. The confidential enquiry into maternal deaths established in 1952 is one example. However, the formalisation of the process with the NHS reforms provided a real impetus to ensure that audit becomes an integral part of clinical work. Some of the basic principles associated with the organisation are perhaps worth restating. Audit should be:

- professionally led;
- seen as an educational process;
- part of routine clinical practice;
- associated with improving quality of care; and
- based on the setting of standards.

The results of audit and the lessons learnt should be disseminated in order to improve care. Health service managers need to be involved in the process and in the outcome of audit.

In some ways, the use of the term 'audit' can be confusing, carrying as it does images of financial audit, a process involving the examination of figures by outside experts. While clinical audit has many forms, at its heart is a critical examination by doctors and other health professionals of their own performance, and comparing this with standards which may be locally or nationally generated, but which are accepted by those carrying out the audit. Thereafter, when audit has shown that change is necessary for the standards to be achieved in practice, these changes must be implemented. Such self scrutiny can be painful, particularly if it highlights poor performance. It is for this reason that so much emphasis is placed on the need for audit to be confidential and carried out by a process in which health professionals have confidence. There is evidence from other countries that where clinical audit has been taken over by some form of inspectorial process, professional energies tend to focus on providing answers that which satisfy the inspector, rather than on genuine self critical examination of their work. Managers in the health service are to be congratulated on the sensitive approach they have taken in allowing the medical profession to develop medical audit over the last three years, and I am confident that the transition to a broader based clinical audit involving other health professionals will also proceed smoothly.

All doctors should be involved in audit, in all specialty groups in hospital, in general practice and in public health. Clinical audit should be seen as a tool for improving care and effecting change, but it is important that it is not seen as a universal way to tackle any question involving professional practice.

This chapter deals with the situation in England, but similar programmes are well developed in Scotland, Wales and Northern Ireland.

Current organisation

At present in England, central funds for clinical audit are disbursed through the regional health authorities, the medical Royal Colleges and other national bodies. Most of the medical audit money for the hospital and community health services has been top-sliced and allocated to the regional health authorities. This has then been disbursed on the advice of the regional medical audit committees to districts and units. Audit for primary care has been built into basic allocations for family health service authorities, and is allocated on the advice of medical audit advisory groups. The Department of Health holds a central fund for the development of audit methods and standards which will be nationally applicable, and for those topics which are appropriate to national audit. Most of this central fund is allocated to the medical Royal Colleges and their Faculties and to other national professional bodies. In 1992–93, £42 million was allocated to audit in the hospital and community health services, £11 million to audit in primary care, and £7 million to nursing and professions allied to medicine. The figures for 1993–94 are even higher — £50.1 million for the development of clinical audit in the hospital and community health services budget (page 139). Over the last few years there has been a great increase in audit activity, with good evidence of changes in clinical practice as a result.*

Regional audit committees are required to submit an annual report on progress, and these committees (regional and local) are the key to the organisation. Until recently, regional audit co-ordinators and their staff met under the auspices of the King's Fund for a series of helpful meetings to discuss practical issues. These meetings have now been formalised and there is an organisational structure related to the Department of Health to deal with practical issues, such as communication between health regions, choice of, and problems with, software, use of the results of audit and so on. This will considerably strengthen the operational aspects of the audit programme.

Almost all the medical Royal Colleges have medical audit or quality of care committees which supervise the programme of work centrally funded by the Department of Health. The work of some of the Colleges is described in Section 2. The audit working

---

*Editor's note: Since Dr Calman wrote this chapter, the Department of Health has issued a circular [EL(93)34] about the integration of medical audit and the audit of other health professionals, and about the future financing of medical audit. This is reproduced as Appendix A on page 139.

group of the Conference of Colleges considers cross-college audit issues, and now meets twice a year with the regional audit co-ordinators group.

Audit and research

There is a continuing debate about the relationship between audit and research, which are clearly related but distinct activities. Audit is about current practice, but research sets out to discover new knowledge. Research will stimulate audit and set new standards; audit will suggest new research ideas. Audit is a quality assurance measure grounded in education, and is essentially comparative. It is about implementation of change, so health service managers and health professionals must work together to achieve changes in practice in delivering health care.

There is a need for a strong science, research and knowledge base for all medical practice. This is the only way in which the results of procedures or treatments and their outcomes can be properly assessed. Finally, there needs to be research into the best methods for audit and the best way to achieve changes in practice.

Some recent developments

The Department of Health has set up the Clinical Outcomes Group, jointly chaired by chief medical and nursing officers, to act as a focus for clinical audit work and to provide overall strategic direction of audit. Four working groups are considering:

- the implications of multiprofessional audit;
- the management aspects of clinical audit;
- the possible need for a clinical audit handbook; and
- the role of guidelines for good practice in clinical work and in audit.

The group's name underlines two particular points. First, *clinical* relates to audit being multiprofessional rather than simply medical. Although there will still be 'medical' projects, 'nursing' projects and so on, the aim is to move towards an integrated approach. Secondly, *outcomes* signals that it is the outcomes of clinical intervention which are important, whether related to the patient, the community, the profession or management. Stressing outcomes does not deny that process is important, but rather that the group's name denotes a shift of the focus of activity.

A look at the future

With these general remarks as a background, what then of the future? Do we have a vision as to how things should develop?

Over the next year, three important areas need to be developed:

- the evolution of uniprofessional audit into multidisciplinary audit;
- the encouragement of an increasing emphasis on the outcomes of care; and
- the greater involvement of managers in the whole audit process.

First, the process of audit should move to become an interprofessional activity, *clinical audit*, as manifest by the title of this book, but it should remain clinically led and educationally based. The move to interprofessional working should take place at a pace with which different professions locally feel comfortable. It is vital that each profession feels that its own audit needs are being catered for, and that the interests of one discipline do not swamp those of another. The confidentiality of the results of audit remains an important principle.

Clinical audit should be seen as part of overall efforts to improve quality. It is the outcome of clinical work or public health measures which should be the focus of activity. In organisational terms, the Clinical Outcomes Group will provide the strategic direction.

There is a need to discuss further the contribution of management to clinical audit. The generation of outcome data will be of little value unless this information can be integrated into management processes. For example, the development of standards and guidelines for care need to become part of the purchasing cycle.

The regional clinical audit co-ordinators should be related to the Clinical Outcomes Group, and the two groups must work closely together. Regional audit representation should broaden to take into account the expertise in audit in all professional groups.

General practice and, more broadly, primary care are areas in which clinical audit particularly needs to be encouraged.

The role of the public in audit needs further discussion. This is not easy, because it is difficult to define who are 'the public'. There needs to be discussion of ways in which public participation might strengthen the importance of the values attached to outcomes when considering the allocation of resources.

Further attention needs to be paid to the introduction of audit into basic, post-graduate, and continuing professional education.

Educational bodies should be asked to outline the part audit plays in the curriculum and in assessment procedures.

Informational aspects of clinical audit need to be developed further, including the development of databases both about available audit protocols and about units undertaking audits on identical or related topics. Better links with research activity are also needed.

Some implications for management

More attention needs to be given to the rights and responsibilities of health service managers in the audit process. These are different for purchaser and provider managers. As far as providers are concerned, trust or unit chief executives have overall responsibility for the care provided within their units, so they must have confidence in the local programme of clinical audit. They should be able to have substantial influence on the content of individual audit programmes, and must be assured that adequate action is taken in response to the findings of audit. Deficiencies revealed by clinical audit more often relate to the running of the organisation than to defective professional practice. The more managers are involved in the whole audit process and its organisation, the more likely that they will be committed to securing the necessary improvements in care highlighted as necessary by the audit process, some of which will inevitably require extra funding. It would be unreasonable for doctors and other health professionals to guard jealously the audit process, and then be disappointed that instant managerial action is not forthcoming in response to audit findings.

Conversely, managers must continue to accept that some aspects of audit are best carried out in confidence, and that inappropriate intrusion will result in the more sensitive areas not being addressed. Local audit committees were devised to protect and manage this delicate interface.

The needs of purchasers are equally important. Clinical audit should be the major plank of the overall quality assurance that purchasers require of the units with which they place contracts. Purchasers have a right to know the arrangements for clinical audit in units and trusts, the level of participation by professional staff, the topics examined and the improvements generated.

The generation of robust outcome data will be of increasing interest and importance to both purchaser and provider managers. Such data should be increasingly linked to the definition of standards and guidelines of care which will need to become part of the overall purchasing cycle. This will all reinforce the importance of involving clinicians directly in discussions between purchasers and providers.

DISCUSSION

Peter Emerson: Dr Calman has talked about the importance of measuring outcome. It is difficult to achieve a robust outcome measure, but one such is mortality rates for surgery. Another is how many of a firm's patients are being operated on by the consultant surgeon and how many by junior staff. Could you give some general guidance about how that sort of data should be disseminated, and who should receive what information about such robust measures? Should it be reported back only to the surgeons concerned, to the physicians in the hospital who have an interest in knowing the mortality rates of their colleagues, or fed to the local community?

Kenneth Calman: I am disappointed that your question implies that this issue has not been discussed locally already, and an answer found. Local audit committees should now be considering how to use the data they collect. I suspect that the decision depends a great deal on the issue. For example, if audit suggests the need for an additional operating theatre or endoscopy suite, and this need is suddenly sprung on the local manager without having involved him or her in the audit, one cannot expect resources to be found immediately.

The measurement of outcomes is a professional issue. It is not for the Department of Health to write down how and what outcomes should be measured. It is for you in clinical practice to develop them, in association with your Colleges or specialist associations.

Section 1

Quality, contract specification and clinical audit

1 | The purchaser's view

Graham Coomber
*formerly District General Manager, North Worcestershire Health
Authority; now Chief Executive, North Birmingham Healthcare
Purchasing Consortium*

As a purchaser, I begin by stating that I do not believe there should
be any incongruence or conflict between the purchaser's and
provider's views of clinical audit.

Medical audit, now subsumed within clinical audit, was defined
in the White Paper[1] as a:

> systematic, critical analysis of the quality of medical care, including the
> procedures used for the diagnosis and treatment, the use of resources
> and the resultant outcome and quality of life for the patient.

The White Paper continued that:

> because a patient's primary concern is for a correct diagnosis to be
> made, and effective treatment to be given, medical audit must be central
> to any programme to enhance the overall quality of care given to patients
> .... An effective programme of medical audit will help provide the neces-
> sary reassurance to doctors, patients and managers that the best possible
> quality of service is being achieved within the resources available.

As a purchaser, my interest is as much in representing the
patient's interests as the manager's, and I need the reassurance
that an effective programme of clinical audit will provide.

The Working Paper accompanying the White Paper also stated
that:

> the Government recognises that medical audit requires commitment
> in terms of clinicians' time, the need for good and accessible medical
> records, adequate information and secretarial staff .... This investment
> will prove worthwhile to both doctors and patients by further improv-
> ing the quality of service offered.[2]

I would have gone further and said that successful clinical audit
requires the total commitment of the organisation.

All these quotations relate specifically to medical audit but, as
virtually all care is given by a multidisciplinary team, they relate to
the audit of care by all health professionals.

At this stage in the development of audit, two questions must be
asked:

- What evidence is there that the investment made in audit so far is providing value for money?
- How many providers can demonstrate to their purchasers that the not inconsiderable investment in audit, in terms of both real and opportunity cost, is worth it, at a time when other costs are being closely scrutinised, and when I, as a purchaser, am demanding 2.5% more activity next year, and giving the providers less money in real terms to do it?

Hopkins and Maxwell reflected that:

A District Health Authority will undoubtedly wish to see audit reports from previous years before placing a contract. It will have to consider the question whether the supplier's audit is something of a decoration or whether it is serious and leads to action.[3]

In short, there is increasingly a need to audit what is going on under the name of audit.*

As a purchaser, I want to know that the audit process is being taken seriously. First, audit is obviously important because it is the only process which can address effectively the evaluation of the clinical care of patients and show how standards and outcomes are being improved.

Secondly, clinical audit is central to the process of quality improvement. In every provider with whom I contract I am look-ing for an organisational culture which is committed to improving quality continually in *everything* that it does. I do not want to have to persuade or cajole providers to take quality improvement seri-ously. If the clinical audit process — the heart of any programme to improve quality — is not being taken seriously, other fine words about commitment to quality are no more than fine words. In short, the state of development of the clinical audit process is a good barometer of the overall health of a provider organisation. Clinical audit is not something which can simply be 'bolted on' to the organisation — it goes to the heart of the way in which the provider is organised.

The following is an extract from one audit report received by my purchasing authority from one of the providers with whom I con-tract:

Audit meetings have been held on a monthly basis; the meetings have been attended by all the medical and nursing staff representatives in

---

*Editor's note: Since Mr Coomber wrote this chapter, the Department of Health has com-missioned Clinical Accountability Services Planning and Evaluation (CASPE) Research to undertake an evaluation of audit. (See, for example, Refs. 4 & 5.)

the department [a surgical speciality]; topics covered during the last 12 months included [a] and [b] .... Discussions about [a certain treatment] following a small study undertaken by one of the SHOs did not reveal any significant difference in the results of individual surgeons. So far audit has not led to any change in service provision, and progress has been hampered by a lack of resources.

Whilst this may not be a typical example, it is fair to say that the reports sent to my purchasing authority do not persuade me that clinical audit is being taken seriously within many provider organisations. Such audit committee reports may of course be selling short what is being undertaken, and it is possible that they are anonymised to the extent that they do not give a true reflection of what is happening. However, to be useful to a purchaser, audit reports should share the output of the process, describe the lessons that have been learnt, the processes that have been changed, and how patient care has been improved.

Improving the effectiveness of clinical audit

Some consultants believe that so far the investment in audit outweighs any benefits that can be demonstrated. As a purchaser, I do not believe that purchasers making specific requirements about audit in contract specifications will make the process more effective, and I am loath to start loading into contracts detailed objectives to be met from the audit process. Clinical audit, and indeed all attempts at improving quality, will fail if audit is just about responding to external imperatives. The Royal Colleges require that the audit process is in place before accrediting training posts, but this does not in itself result in effective audit. The responsibility for achieving successful audit lies with the providers of health care. How can this commitment be brought about? We need a culture in which everyone is committed to improving their part of the organisation all the time. It is not good enough to have an organisation that works on the principle that 'if it ain't broke, don't fix it'. We need a culture in which it is recognised that by understanding and learning from our mistakes we can move forward. Failure should not result in a witch-hunt and punishment of the guilty, but in the realisation that things go wrong when processes or systems fail.

In managerial life, there is much emphasis and pride on being 'results-orientated'. Some of our management systems, such as individual performance review, drive us that way. No people could care more about the end results of their work than the Japanese, but they understand only too well that it is the processes operating within the organisation that determine the quality of those end results. We need a culture in which clinicians and managers trust each other, and feel confident that together they can act upon the results of audit to improve the systems and processes of care.

Conclusion

From the purchaser's perspective, I need to know that the audit process by my providers is serious, and is leading to action. The only requirement I make when specifying contracts is that I should receive the annual report of the audit committee. This should tell me what I need to know — but the report must do justice to what is going on under the name of audit.

Developing an appropriate organisational culture in which quality is valued has to be the proper business of providers. Purchasers need to support the providers in this process. If there are short-term costs of implementation, purchasers must commit themselves to work with providers in supporting that implementation. Purchasers also need to understand and be sensitive to the issues, and to realise that the further development of clinical audit is a long-term process.

References

1. Department of Health. *Working for Patients*. London: HMSO, 1989
2. Department of Health. *Working Paper No. 6*. London: HMSO, 1989 (accompanying Reference 1)
3. Hopkins A, Maxwell R. *British Medical Journal* 1990: **300**: 922–5
4. Walshe K, Coles J. *Evaluating audit: a review of initiatives*. London: CASPE Research, 1993
5. Walshe K, Coles J. *Evaluating audit: developing a framework*. London: CASPE Research, 1993

2 | The provider's view

Derek Smith
Chief Executive, King's Healthcare NHS Trust

I use the experience of clinical audit gained in my hospital (King's College Hospital) to illustrate the provider's perspective of audit, and the effect of competitive pressures on audit.

Three themes characterise clinical audit at the hospital:

- it is multidisciplinary in nature;
- it is as integral to management as it is to the care of patients; and
- there remains a lack of clarity between purchasers and providers about that which is to be audited. This needs urgent resolution.

Clinical audit has developed more quickly in the specialties in which there is already competition and risk than in other specialties not facing the same levels of competitive pressure.

The multidisciplinary approach which has been adopted is demonstrated by the structure of the clinical audit committee (Table 1). The first chair was the Professor of Medicine. He has been succeeded by another doctor, and thereafter, a member of another profession may chair the committee.

The common difficulty is that audit committees were initially district based, yet as units became separate NHS Trusts they needed to build their own audit structure. This has not applied at King's as the Trust originally incorporated all the services provided by the Camberwell District Health Authority in April 1992. If anything,

Table 1. Composition of King's Healthcare clinical audit committee

Chair	3 Representatives of education (medical, dental, nursing)
Vice chair	
Audit co-ordinator	1 Profession allied to medicine
Member of trust board	1 Senior manager
5 Doctors (including 1 junior)	3 Customers (purchaser, patient's advocate, general practitioner representative)
3 Nurses	

difficulties at King's concerning audit have centred upon the establishment of 'medical' and 'nursing' audit at regional level, and upon national direction which has channelled funding streams in separate directions. (These arrangements have since been superseded by a multidisciplinary approach nationwide.)

Formal accountability of the committee to the trust board is through the executive director, nursing. The committee has to produce an annual report, but the board has also established a subcommittee comprising non-executive and executive members which is concerned with all aspects of service quality. A concept of a 'quality framework' has been developed (Fig. 1), to which clinical audit is a principal contributor.

The clinical audit approach has been used to pursue management as well as clinical objectives. One example is related to the sickle-cell service. There were specific concerns about the type of service being offered, some of which were expressed by service providers and users. The authority given under circular HC(91)2[1]

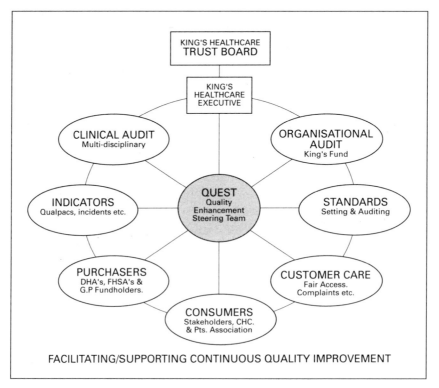

Fig 1. *Dimensions of service quality and lines of accountability — King's Healthcare.*

was used to ask the clinical audit committee to study aspects of our care of this disorder, not only in relation to the clinical aspects but also to behavioural and cultural concerns about the care provided. The result of the audit is agreement on the most effective clinical regimen, and a costed plan of action. Without a multidisciplinary approach, this many-faceted matter could not have been resolved.

There has been a lack of consistency between purchaser and provider as to what should be audited in the first place. The South-East London Commissioning Agency had its own priorities for audit, but only 50% of these accorded with the King's Healthcare clinical audit plan. Complementary audit plans need to be established which meet the mutual needs of both purchaser and provider. Such plans will have to be constructed with the involvement of clinical staff of all disciplines at an early stage, and will require negotiation between the organisations concerned. However, where there is room both for competition, with the risk of service shifts from one provider to another and also for difference between the aims of purchasers and of providers, there is unlikely to be 100% agreement on the priorities for audit.* Clinicians and providers will also baulk at purchasers attempting to set the agenda, if they take the view that public health expertise is less informed than clinical expertise in the specifics of treatment and care.

The interests of purchasers and providers do however coincide over money. Until 5 April 1995, funding of medical and nursing audit will be 'ring-fenced', so that funds cannot be diverted to other priorities. In future, purchasers will have to consider the trade-off between the amount of health care interventions to be bought and the steps that should be taken towards enhancing quality.[2]

The relationship between buyers and sellers in the managed health care market becomes different if there is a degree of competition. King's Healthcare operates on two sites in London, not far south of the river. Guy's, St Thomas's, St George's and Lewisham Hospitals are nearby. Our main commissioning health authority and several of those which are significant contractors are all losing funding through weighted capitation. The report of the London Implementation Group[3] will result in major planned service changes for inner London. In these circumstances, will the provider be enthusiastic about informing the purchaser about service quality, which may not attain the performance of competitors? For example, for

---

*A new audit structure has since been proposed for South East Thames, partly to achieve a consistent approach between purchasers and providers.

many years cardiothoracic surgeons have maintained a register enabling crude comparisons of survival rates. Now, however, the Parsonnet score, derived from a risk stratification based upon the age and condition of the patient, can be used to help compare the outcomes of surgery.[4] Purchasers have not yet used such information to adjust their purchasing patterns, but the information is available for them to move from a dialogue about price and service volume to a comparison of outcomes, and to place contracts accordingly.

Such improved information may create another problem for hospital managers. What if there are significant differences in outcome from surgeon to surgeon? Failure to act could leave patients at a higher risk than necessary and damage the reputation of the cardiac unit, leaving it prey to reductions in contract size. To act is likely to damage the livelihood and professional reputation of any surgeon who is demonstrably achieving less good outcomes than colleagues, even though his or her results may be no worse than surgeons practising in other parts of the country.

Competition has driven clinicians to explore the legitimate boundaries of practice. We plan to reduce the use of intensive therapy at King's for post-operative cardiovascular surgery patients by 50% in 1993–94 and by 20–25% in 1994–95. The consequences for patients must be assessed, and so a prospective audit will be conducted. In the related area of angioplasty, more patients are being treated, where previously they were scheduled for coronary artery bypass grafts. This has the beneficial effect for patients of reducing the time spent waiting for treatment, and of course makes the service itself more competitive. The overriding question is whether percutaneous transluminal coronary angioplasty will lead to at least as good an outcome as a coronary artery bypass graft. Clinical audit will enable us to study the outcomes and to test whether this approach to coronary artery disease will have a genuine benefit for patients themselves.*

The cardiac unit is taking a broadly based approach to improving its service quality. Nurses are active in evaluating rehabilitation practice and the benefits of health education for cardiac patients. Clinical audit cannot be just about winning and losing in the market-place. It must be born of a genuine commitment by those providing care to seek improvements in the service they offer. Competitive advantage will accrue as a by-product of good care and the use of audit to sustain improvements.

---

*Editor's note: Such questions are better answered by research studies than by audit, and indeed the Randomised Intervention Treatment of Angina (RITA) trial has already provided some answers to the questions posed.[5]

References

1. Department of Health. *Medical Audit in the Hospital and Community Health Services: Assuring the Quality of Medical Care; Implementation of Medical and Dental Audit.* Circular HC(91)2. London: Department of Health, 1991
2. Department of Health. *Clinical audit in HCHS: allocation of funds 1993/94.* Circular HC(93)34. London: Department of Health, 1993 (reproduced as Appendix A)
3. Tomlinson B. Report of the inquiry into London's health service, medical education and research. London: HMSO, 1992
4. Parsonnet V, Dean D, Bernstein AD. A method of uniform stratification of risk for evaluating the results of surgery in acquired adult heart disease. *Circulation* 1989; **701** (suppl): 13–113
5. Randomised Intervention Treatment of Angina trial participants. Coronary angioplasty versus coronary artery bypass surgery: the Randomised Intervention Treatment of Angina (RITA) trial. *Lancet* 1993; **341**: 573–80

3 | New relationships between general practitioner fundholders and hospital clinicians

David Colin-Thome
General Practitioner, Runcorn, Cheshire

The first two years of fundholding have probably seen an undue concentration on the purchasing of secondary care. This aspect of fundholding has without doubt been one of the key factors in changing secondary care behaviour, as hospitals have become much more responsive to patients' and general practitioners' needs.

The main attraction of fundholding for our practice was the acquisition of a primary care budget that we ourselves can manage. Purchasing hospital care has been an important but secondary consideration. The emphasis on a primary care budget puts pressure on general practitioners to provide good quality local services, some of which can — but need not — be purchased from the hospital, thereby blurring the interface between primary and secondary care.

For our first two years of hospital purchasing, three themes were developed:

- referral activity should reflect the needs of patients;
- different types of contracts are appropriate for different clinical disorders and different provider units (eg block, cost and volume, or cost per case contracts); and
- contracts should contain specifications of quality that reflect the perspectives of the users of the services.

In the first year of fundholding there was little contact with hospital consultants, mainly because of the antipathy of some of them to the new world. We had previously worked with some local consultants in writing joint protocols for certain diseases, so to some extent the National Health Service (NHS) reforms set back these relationships.

Prior to fundholding, a postal consumer survey of our services had been undertaken involving 10% of our practice population.

This received an encouraging 53% response, despite the proforma taking some 20 minutes to complete. The survey was undertaken independently of the practice, and some intriguing questions were asked, such as, 'Did the doctor listen to you?', and 'Did the doctor address the problem with which you went?'. In response to some negative replies to these questions, our counsellor reviewed video recordings of consultations, thus giving a different perspective of our performance — a non-medical member of the team influencing a key aspect of patient care. Patient access to our services was also increased as a result of the survey.

The practice partners have for some years audited one another's consultations by reviewing clinical aspects of care, but the advent of a fundholding budget provided the necessary impetus to undertake more audit, so as to be more effective resource managers. Audits are presented at the fortnightly partners' meeting which is sometimes attended by hospital staff. Over 70% generic prescribing had already been achieved even prior to the practice becoming fundholding. Clinical audit has shown that, as a group, we can respond to practice guidelines with changes in prescribing habits, and consequent further savings on our prescribing budget. An audit of treatment of asthma, for example, revealed that in the past bronchodilators were prescribed more than three times as often as steroids. The balance is now nearly equal, as recommended.[1] This particular change has increased our prescribing costs, but it is felt that we are giving the best treatment by responding to national guidelines. However, the costs of prescribing have been reduced in other areas such as non-steroidal anti-inflammatory agents and antibiotics. About one-third of the prescribing budget is outside our control, insofar as cancer chemotherapy, some appliances, insulin and so on are very much part of hospital practice, and there is a need to work more closely with hospital colleagues in this area.

Dietetic and musculo-skeletal physiotherapy services for the practice are currently contracted with the hospital, and these services have been audited. The dietetic audit was concerned only with organisational audit, but the service has become more cost-effective by reducing the number of non-attenders. The physiotherapy audit revealed inappropriate referrals by general practitioners. The physiotherapist was asked to train us in the best management of back problems, and she reviewed the appropriateness of her follow-up of certain conditions. As a result of such joint working, new orthopaedic referrals are now 20% less than the pattern established over previous years.

A review of surgical outpatient referrals was undertaken as it is our

most frequent and costly service. The outcome of our patients' attendances with the surgeons was looked at, focusing on the appropriateness of referral. In 1991, 60% of referrals resulted in surgical 'interventions', in the sense that an operation was carried out or a surgical
diagnosis made; 25% of patients were reassured, and in 15% the
referral 'failed' insofar as the patient failed to attend, the referral
was to the wrong specialty, or an operation requested by the general
practitioner was considered not necessary. In 1992, after the audit,
the relevant percentages were 71%, 19% and 10%. Practice partners
now undertake much more minor surgery, as a result of which the
percentage of patients referred has fallen by 14%, and the rate for
failed attendance by those referred has fallen from 30% to 5%.

The most expensive investigations requested are those carried
out in the X-ray department. Our X-ray requests have fallen by
30% in the last two years. The open-access gastroscopy service, for
which long waiting lists had developed, has also been audited,
which resulted in a review of our approach to gastroscopy referrals.
With the help of local consultants, an open-access colonoscopy service has also been initiated, thus cutting out unnecessary outpatient attendances. This approach followed a hospital audit on rec-
tal bleeding, an excellent example of primary and secondary care
working together. Much of this work in radiology, gastroscopy and
surgery will influence how services are purchased next year.

For some time a full range of mental health workers has been
working at the practice. We employ our own counsellor and have
the benefit of two sessions of clinical psychology and one of community psychiatric nursing per week. As a result, referrals to adult
psychiatry clinics are only about 50 patients per year for a practice
population of 12,000.

A part-time information manager has been employed so that our
fully computerised practice can use the computer as an audit tool
to save time and effort. The information manager is currently
comparing year-on-year variations in glycosylated haemoglobin in
diabetic patients and peak flow rates of asthmatic patients, to audit
the effectiveness of our clinics. These are early and certainly
incomplete instruments of measurement of outcome, but we
expect to progress to measuring other outcomes of care. The practice is also involved in a joint project with the community health
services unit to audit referral patterns to community services and
their response. Finally, together with purchasing managers, other
general practitioners, public health physicians and hospital consultants, we are writing guidelines for good practice in order to write
contracts appropriately.

Clinical audit has also helped identify the training needs of the partners. For example, audit showed that I had an exceptionally high referral rate to orthopaedic surgeons and for spinal X-rays. As a result of the audit and of discussion with hospital colleagues about the appropriateness of referral for various conditions, my referral rate now approximates to that of my partners.

General practitioners often feel pressed by the volume of their work, and some may feel that audit is just another burden. However, I would say that audit, by concentrating our minds on what we *should* be doing, may release time both for audit and for better practice.

The fundholding general practitioner, as both purchaser and provider, and yet also clinician, should be the link between the service and the patient to enable best care.

Reference

1. British Thoracic Society, British Paediatric Association, Research Unit of the Royal College of Physicians of London, King's Fund Centre, National Asthma Campaign, Royal College of General Practitioners, General Practitioners in Asthma Group, British Association of Accident and Emergency Medicine, British Paediatric Respiratory Group. Guidelines on the management of asthma. *Thorax* 1993: **48**: S1–S24

DISCUSSION

Christopher Tallents: First, how many of us feel that quality is equated with cost? Clearly it may be possible to drive costs down, but at which point does practice become cloned to mediocrity? The second question is a much more sensitive one for consultants. They become increasingly rigid in professional terms as they reach their mid-50s, and there is no real method in this country — and no resources — by which a consultant who wishes to retrain adequately into a new area of work can do so. Should the audit resource be able to provide that sort of funding?

David Colin-Thome: Professionals are driven by values, and they set standards to achieve the best quality. Fundholding general practitioners can manage their budget to shift resources in an imaginative way. There may be a time when we run out of cash, of course, and priorities will then have to be set, but so far it has been possible to increase expenditure, particularly extra nursing care, because of our under-spend in other audited areas.

Derek Smith: I think there is a finite limit to the extent to which costs can be driven down. If we take the example of Japanese cars, they are not cheap, but they are good value and a high quality product. In a sense, this is what we are looking for also in health care. No-one envisages the costs being driven down indefinitely.

Graham Coomber: One problem is that we tend to focus on the costs of improving quality, and are not so good at recognising the costs of 'non-conformance to standards', to use a term from industry. Studies in industry have shown just how much poor quality really costs. We should be more sensitive to the costs of poor quality care, both to our patients and to our organisations.

Leslie Turnberg: We all talk about quality, but at present there are largely only qualitative judgements of quality. As Anthony Hopkins has discussed elsewhere,[1,2] these need to be made quantitative.

Leora Schachter: Do you envisage a situation developing in which audit will allow a more cost-effective choice of provider to be identified?

David Colin-Thome: I see that as the way forward. Why involve doctors in purchasing unless they look at the quality of clinical care? Sometimes we want to look at the views and practices of different consultants which might influence our purchasing in the future, and consultants visit the practice. There are enough referrals to consultants to make this a worthwhile use of resources. Furthermore, they help us set standards by sharing experiences.

Leora Schachter: Whose audit should we believe? Should we listen to our local specialists or another group of doctors who do not have a specialist expertise in the area under review, but are looking at clinical work from outside, driven by budgetary considerations?

David Colin-Thome: I believe that peer review is the way to start, because it is the least threatening. Once confidence in that approach is gained, we will have the confidence to share our work with outside people. Already, our audit is shared with other general practitioners in the group which I have formed, as well as with some non-medical colleagues. It is just a matter of confidence and building relationships so that we start sharing our audit externally, in a more imaginative way.

Leslie Turnberg: Respiratory physicians have set up their own audit system whereby respiratory physicians from one health region visit respiratory units in another, auditing each other's activities and making suggestions for improving clinical practice.*

Alan Amias: My experience at St George's Hospital is that the presence of a majority of clinicians from different specialities has driven the process forward, and encouraged the development of audit in

*Editor's note: Anyone interested in this scheme should consult Dr Brian Harrison, a respiratory physician at Norwich, or the British Thoracic Society.

different directorates. The professional and educational aspects of audit are still prominent in our minds, yet the constitution of the committee at St George's does not seem to reflect these priorities.

Derek Smith: There were initially more consultants on the committee at King's Healthcare, but it was decided that it should develop into more of a steering body. Audit had already developed in most significant clinical departments and services. The present membership of the committee may reflect a further stage of development. No doubt the committee will itself examine its structure, and perhaps choose to change in the future. We believe that it is now mature and developed enough, in terms of our organisation, to be able to look after itself.

Richard Wray: As the wishes of general practitioners are increasingly taken into account within the hospital, a practical problem is beginning to emerge. If fifty or more practices refer to one provider unit, the justifiable protocols based on the interests and expertise of particular general practitioners are leading to a complex situation. Consultants have to check who has sent whom, and whether they are in possession of an up-to-date practice protocol about what the referring general practitioner wants. Could you address the sheer practicalities of this situation?

David Colin-Thome: I can speak only for our own approach. It is not specified in the contracts what consultants are expected to do, because we think that interferes far too much with detailed clinical activity. We say that we would like to discuss how we handle the patients before referring them. We would then be in a position to say to a consultant, 'We have done so-and-so, and we believe this patient might have such-and-such', or 'For your opinion, but the following investigations have been undertaken'. Some of those investigations would have been discussed and agreed between consultants and general practitioners earlier.

We want to use the changes induced by the NHS reforms to focus our attention on the use of this resource rather than duplicating investigations and so on, as in the old days.

Another example is related to the management of high blood pressure. It is generally accepted that three blood pressure readings, each above a certain threshold, should be obtained before starting treatment. However, many patients are started on treatment, some at least unnecessarily, after just one reading. The development of guidelines through central and local joint educative approaches, rather than specifying detailed approaches in contracts, has provided the incentive to work well.

Richard Wray: In Hastings, we are just beginning to get different protocols from different general practitioners, which I think is to be expected. The standard of general practice in our locality is high, and it is a natural development that general practitioners will wish to play a full part in determining what investigations are done and how care is to be provided. This is to be welcomed, but there is some impracticality in multiple linkages, and it is not easy to remember with which linkage we are dealing when managing an individual patient.

Anthony Hopkins: The power of research is important here. It is anomalous that a small group of general practitioners or hospital consultants in isolation should decide what *ought* to be done — whether in Hastings, Manchester, or anywhere else. The evidence for what ought to be done must be found from the research litera-ture. If research has determined which patients require an X-ray after a head injury, for example, it is wasteful of resources for gener-al practitioners or hospital consultants to suggest other criteria with-out equally good or better *research* evidence. As another example, in response to the questionnaire described in Chapter 20, a colleague said that audit had shown that a second review colposcopy after a biopsy for intra-epithelial carcinoma of the cervix was unnecessary, and that his unit had changed its practice. This sounds fine — but such policies ought not to be decided by an audit of forty or fifty cases, however well intentioned. Such a question has to be decided by careful multicentre controlled trials, which set the standard, and only then do we move on to clinical audit.

Enormous gaps in the research literature are emerging from a critical appraisal of what is available. These allow the development of a whole raft of potentially ill-prepared guidelines. Some criteria need to be developed by which the validity and value of individual guidelines are determined.*

Ann Edwards: In what appears to be an increasingly cost-led system for providing medical care, is it visualised that clinical audit will take a prime role in maintaining integration of the system, for the benefit of the patients?

**Graham Winyard: I do not accept that we will be cost-led, as opposed to being cost-conscious. Anthony Hopkins pointed out that in many areas of practice it is uncertain as to what should be done. There are other areas in which, while best practice has been defined, such practice is not being followed. This is the importance

---

*Editor's note: Since this discussion the NHS Management Executive has commissioned the development of appraisal criteria for clinical guidelines.
**Editor's note: Shortly after this meeting, Graham Winyard was appointed Deputy Chief Medical Officer and Medical Director of the NHS Management Executive.

of clinical audit: there will undoubtedly be areas where cost restrictions prevent clinicians from delivering the best care, and these need to be drawn to the attention of managers and of local public health physicians so that attempts can be made to improve the situation and, if necessary, more resources obtained. At the same time, good audit will discover ways in which resources, which are inevitably limited, can be better used.

Patrick Jeffery: Purchasers have a legitimate interest in driving the activities of the audit committee, but that committee needs to retain ownership of its activities, drive itself, and take notice of what goes on regionally. I had the impression from Mr Coomber's presentation that he was interested in dictating — but *diktats* get us nowhere. There has to be dialogue, discussion and mutual agreement. How does he, as a purchaser, see that process happening?

Graham Coomber: I may have misled you. We are not talking about a *diktat*. Clinical audit seems to be a classic case for a joint purchaser-provider approach, but it worries me greatly if, as Derek Smith mentioned (although I do not know his local situation) there are different perspectives, and purchasers and providers are driving audit in different directions. There will obviously be differences, but it ought to be possible to agree a mostly common agenda.

David Colin-Thome: One of my concerns is that we do not become obsessed by new structures. Even though some sort of structure is needed, a lot of audit activity is driven by such questions as what sort of committee to set up, rather than it being part of the natural process of professionals simply undertaking audit.

Graham Winyard: There is evidence from other countries of a danger that, if there is too much of an inspectorial approach to audit from heavy handed purchasers, and if too many questions are pressed via the clinical audit route, the energies of those being audited are directed to satisfying the questions rather than to being self critical.

The other danger is that of using clinical audit as an all-purpose tool to address any issue about clinical care. Purchasers are fully entitled to ask searching questions of the provider units with which they are placing contracts, but it should be up to those units to decide how they provide the answers. Very often this will form some method other than clinical audit.

References

1. Hopkins A. *Measuring the quality of medical care.* London: Royal College of Physicians of London, 1990
2. Hopkins A. Costain D eds. *Measuring the outcomes of medical care.* London: Royal College of Physicians of London, 1990

Section 2

What some of the Royal Colleges are doing in relation to clinical audit

4 | Royal College of General Practitioners

Michael Pringle
Professor of General Practice, University of Nottingham

The Royal College of General Practitioners' audit programme is a three-year programme which started in April 1990, comprising four strands: education, gathering information, development, and the dissemination of information about audit. There is a related programme of research which is not part of the audit programme itself but which is being undertaken by the College as a separate venture.

The College has set up a series of courses available to general practitioners and to those working in audit in general practice throughout the United Kingdom. These are usually fully subscribed.

The College also runs seminars and sessions for the chairmen of the medical audit advisory groups throughout the United Kingdom and for their audit facilitators. The latter have been identified as a key group for the College's audit activity. Members of these groups are often ill-supported, and value the College's contribution. With regard to gathering information, the College maintains a central database of audit literature and activity, and a register of people with particular interests.

The development programme has involved the appointment of four audit fellows throughout the country (Mersey, Tamar, the North of England and North-West London). The projects of these audit fellows were designed as demonstration, torch-bearing projects, which could show the rest of general practice what was potentially achievable in their areas. Unlike many other specialties, it is not realistic in general practice to run a nationwide, all-encompassing audit from the centre. The Mersey audit fellow, for example, is developing interpractice audits in such areas as terminal care, deaths in the practice, benzodiazepine withdrawal, alcohol problems and care for patients with schizophrenia. In Tamar, the audit fellow offers a menu of different audits to all the practices in the area. Practices have signed up for those that they particularly wish to do, and their results have then been compared. They are now on their fifth round of such audits, having been offered as many as

20 different choices. In the North of England, the audit fellow has concentrated on the educational and structural aspects of audit, and helped to co-ordinate the medical audit advisory groups and evaluate audit methodology. In North-West London, the audit fellow has developed a database of local activity, and provided packaged audit protocols for participating practices.

One of these schemes has been less successful than the other three, but overall we believe that they have shown a way forward for practices and for areas in the country to co-ordinate audit activity and to begin to relate not just single practice audits to the wide context but also to compare practices and gain an understanding of what is happening in a wider sense.

The College is also involved in a number of collaborative projects across interprofessional boundaries. Multidisciplinary audits are being undertaken with pathologists, midwives and orthopaedic and general surgeons.

A major initiative has been to identify the terms and concepts used in medical audit in general practice and to try to codify them into some sort of thesaurus. A publication entitled, *Meanings and medical audit*, will be published by the College later in 1994. An audit enquiry service and a 'newsline' are also run.

The College is exploring some key issues believed to be important for the development of medical audit as an academic discipline within primary care. Audit is dependent upon the information systems that practices have available, some of which have severe shortfalls with regard to medical audit. For example, 70% of all computer systems cannot measure the continuity of care offered to patients — a measure that might be regarded as a fundamental index of the care offered by a practice.

A study by the College comparing the relative values of case-based and cohort audit is nearing completion.

Lastly, the College has been looking at the audit activity within a sample of practices, to explore the changes in attitudes over the last two years. It is gratifyingly high in a large number of practices, but a small minority of practices have yet to start *any* audit activity. Attitudes to audit among general practitioners are improving and, as might be expected, those who get involved in audit change their attitudes more positively with time.

Audit activity must be demonstrated to lead to improvement in quality of care. As yet, there is no firm evidence to justify all the audit activity which is going on. It is a matter of faith and belief with us that audit *will* improve patient care, but we have a responsibility to demonstrate that link.

5 | Royal College of Psychiatrists

Paul Lelliott
Research Unit, Royal College of Psychiatrists

An audit working group, chaired by the Registrar of the Royal College of Psychiatrists, produced the initial guidelines for audit in psychiatry.[1] The College's main audit programme, like that of the Royal College of Physicians, is centred on the College Research Unit which is entering its third year of audit work, funded by the Department of Health.

The audit programme reflects the College's belief in the wider function of audit in the changing health service, which endorses the importance of audit in informing management and purchasing processes as well as the work of clinical psychiatrists.

In addition to medical and clinical audit, which focus on the clinical activities of the psychiatrist and the teams within which they work, the College added 'service planning audit' and 'needs-based audit'.

Service planning audit measures the extent to which a mental health service delivers appropriate care to those that use it, often through the evaluation of how a service is currently being used. The information derived informs managers (who, in mental health services, are increasingly clinicians) both about future planning and about the effect that previous decisions have had on patient care. Service planning audit is therefore part of resource management.

Needs-based audit measures the extent to which a service meets the needs of its catchment population, and includes issues of outreach and identification of unmet need. Audit thus has a role in informing purchasing authorities of the nature and quantity of services which they should be purchasing for their catchment population. This is particularly appropriate for modern psychiatric services which are now more often organised to provide services to a geographically-defined catchment area (the 'sector').

The aims of the Research Unit of the College are to assist in the development of *clinical standards* and to review the *structure of services* required for general psychiatry and psychiatric specialties, including advice on the epidemiological characteristics of higher- and lower-needs districts. The Research Unit also provides *information and advice* on audit, and provides advice for, and collaborates in initiatives on *mental health information systems.* The collection and delivery of good information underpins audit.

One of the first tasks was to establish a line of communication with local mental health services, so a national survey of psychiatric audit activity was undertaken.[2] There is now a register of psychiatrists who are taking the lead in audit in over 90% of districts and health boards in the United Kingdom. This register has been used both to communicate the work of the unit and to recruit mental health services into multicentre audit projects.

Audit projects

Audit projects set up by the College include:

1. *Setting clinical standards*

    Twelve years ago, Dr. John Pippard conducted a national survey of electroconvulsive therapy (ECT) practice,[3] on the basis of which the College published recommendations on the conduct of the administration of ECT.[4] Two years ago, the Research Unit asked Dr Pippard to repeat the survey in two health regions to audit the impact of the guidelines. The results showed that, while some aspects of practice had improved, some had not, in particular the training and supervision given to junior doctors administering ECT.[5]

    This posed a challenge, in that producing recommendations had been insufficient by themselves to bring about change. A special committee was established to consider these findings, and their implications. As a result, the College organised a series of educational workshops through its programme of continuing medical education, which are aimed at reaching all consultants responsible for supervising ECT in local districts. A further multisite survey is planned to gauge the effectiveness of this further action.

2. *A confidential enquiry into homicides and suicides:*

    The College has used the Research Unit's register of audit convenors to recruit districts into this project, which was established in collaboration with the Department of Health. About 150 districts (about three-quarters of the then national total) have responded, and about 80 recently attended a symposium, at which this audit was launched. Information about homicides and suicides will be collated by the College in a way analogous to the Confidential Enquiry into Perioperative Deaths (CEPOD).[6]

3. *An audit of acute admissions of those mentally ill*
   A survey of admissions and discharges to two inner London acute psychiatric units (Camberwell and Riverside) has been completed, affording an overview of the quality of care provided by two inner-city acute psychiatric units. It indicates reasons for admissions, identifies support (had it been available) that might have prevented admission, and illustrates some of the problems caused by heavy pressure on beds and resulting high bed occupancy rates.

   The preliminary findings have been made available to the services concerned. The intention is to repeat the audit after the implementation of the new community care arrangements, in order to assess their effects on the use of acute wards.

4. *An audit of new long-stay psychiatric patients*
   Fifty-nine services in the United Kingdom have provided information on the characteristics and needs for care of all patients in their catchment areas who have been admitted in the past three years and who have been inpatients for more than six months, thus identifying patients who could not be discharged despite the current focus on community care. This survey provides information on which planning can be made for the needs of this group of particularly disadvantaged patients, and also provides a baseline for monitoring the impact of implementation of the community care legislation outlined in *Caring for people*,[7] the findings of the Reed Committee[8] and the Tomlinson report.[9] In one district (Cambridge) the survey has been extended to patients resident in all forms of accommodation, including local authority and the voluntary sector. This has piloted an approach that would give an epidemiological base to assessing districts needs for provision for this group of patients.[10]

Information and advice on audit

The College has established an Audit and Information Technology office, the role of which includes the dissemination of the results of the audit work of the College and its Research Unit and responding to enquiries from all sources on audit issues.

Mental health information systems

Good quality clinical information is a necessary prerequisite for audit. There is evidence that existing information systems are failing adequately to support clinical care — and therefore audit.[11] The Research Unit has been an essential contributor to the College's involvement in recent initiatives in mental health informatics. It serviced a mental health information systems working group,[12] which drafted a minimal clinical data set for discussion, and reviewed existing systems against functional requirements.[13]

The Director of the Research Unit (Professor John Wing) is the College's representative on the working group on information technology of the Conference of Colleges, and chairman of the speciality working group developing Read codes for psychiatry through the Clinical Terms Project. As part of a separate project, brief outcome scales, usable in clinical practice, are being developed and piloted. These initiatives will facilitate the evolution of audit of outcomes as opposed to that of structure and process.

References

1. Gath A. Audit. *Psychiatric Bulletin* 1991; **15**: 23-25
2. Lelliott P. *Clinical audit in psychiatry. Hospital Update.* 1994; (in press)
3. Pippard J, Ellam L. Electroconvulsive treatment in Great Britain. *British Journal of Psychiatry* 1981; **139**: 563-8
4. Royal College of Psychiatrists. *The practical administration of electroconvulsive therapy.* London: Gaskell, 1989
5. Pippard J. Audit of electroconvulsive treatment in two NHS Regions. *British Journal of Psychiatry* 1992; **160**: 621-37
6. Campling EA, Devlin HB, Hoile RW, Lunn JN. *The report of the national Confidential Enquiry into Perioperative Deaths* 1991/2. London: NCEPOD Royal College of Surgeons 1993
7. Department of Health: *Caring for people: community care in the next decade and beyond.* London: HMSO, 1989
8. Department of Health and Home Office. *Review of health and social services for mentally disordered offenders and others requiring similar services.* (Reed J, chmn). London: HMSO, 1992
9. Tomlinson B. *Inquiry into London's health service, medical education and research.* London: HMSO, 1992
10. Wing J. *Epidemiologically-based mental health needs assessment.* Oxford: Radcliffe, 1994 (in press)
11. Audit Commission. *Caring Systems: A handbook for managers of nursing and project managers.* London: HMSO, 1992
12. Mental health information systems working group: *Report to the Research Committee.* London: Royal College of Psychiatrists, (Available from the Research Unit of the RCPsych, 17 Belgrave Square, London SW1X 8PG) 1992
13. Lelliott P, Flannigan C, Shanks S. *A review of seven mental health information systems: A functional perspective.* London: Research Unit Publications 1, Royal College of Psychiatrists, 1993

6 | Royal College of Surgeons of England

David Dunn
Consultant Surgeon, Addenbrooke's Hospital, Cambridge

The Royal College of Surgeons of England is active in the field of audit under the leadership of Mr Brendan Devlin, chairman of the College's Audit Committee. Table 1 illustrates some of the projects being undertaken, but this does not include other major initiatives, such as the National Confidential Enquiry into Perioperative Deaths, (NCEPOD),[1] our publications on audit, or the various road-shows and meetings about audit organised by the College for audit co-ordinators and assistants, nurses, junior doctors, managers and delegates from industry. Almost all the activities described by representatives of other Colleges are also going on at the Royal College of Surgeons. Most of the projects listed in Table 1 have research fellows appointed to run them. They undertake individual audits of various aspects of surgical care, including patient satisfaction.

Audit Projects

I will describe two projects briefly, to illustrate the pattern they

Table 1. Surgical audit projects

- Management of ankle fractures
- Upper gastrointestinal endoscopy
- Prostatectomy
- Management of colorectal cancer
- Management of cleft lip and palate
- Patient satisfaction survey
- Development of patient information leaflets
- Management of groin hernia in adults
- Audit of day surgery
- Audit of liver transplant services
- Audit of anticoagulant therapy
- Management of upper gastrointestinal haemorrhage
- Confidential comparative audit service

follow, and then discuss the confidential comparative audit service in more detail as this is different from what other Colleges have been doing.

Fracture of the ankle

First, the management of ankle fractures. Details on 1,000 ankle fractures have been collected throughout the country, analysed, and their management critically appraised. A report and practice guidelines are in preparation.

Upper gastrointestinal endoscopy

In conjunction with some other Royal Colleges, over 14,000 endoscopies have been studied. Data on safety and patient monitoring have been analysed, and attempts made to assess the appropriate use of endoscopy, and patient satisfaction. Overall mortality figures have been derived and a report is in press.

The comparative audit service

Audit in surgery, which the College has stimulated in the ways mentioned above, occurs locally in the surgical units. This is where surgeons collect data, look at their patients, review their complication rates, and make recommendations which complete the audit cycle. Many surgeons now have good data collection systems as part of their work, which make audit data easily available and local audit meetings relatively easy to run. However, it is difficult to know what such local results mean without other results with which they can be compared. The scientific literature provides some comparisons, but these usually seem to emanate from a pristine hospital with excellent results, which appear not to relate to the hospitals of local surgeons where many patients are elderly and suffer from serious disease and comorbidity. Furthermore, published papers are often written several years prior to the current audit. A contemporary comparison is required to see whether local results are out of line, and to highlight areas in which action is needed.

The comparative audit service of the College was set up in 1991 to provide surgeons with such comparisons. Proformas are sent to local surgeons who fill in a data set which the College considers to be the minimum necessary for the comparison of one surgical practice with another. The results are correlated and analysed, and the comparisons fed back to the individual surgeons, informing them where they stand in relation to this large database. Table 2 shows the numbers of general surgeons contacted in 1990 and 1991 and those who have returned data. Many consultants are not able to get hold of the required data because those data do not exist either in their hospital data systems or in their own records. This explains, in part, the response rate of only 21%. So far 388,000 admissions and 295,000 procedures have been analysed.

Table 2. Royal College of Surgeons comparative audit service: numbers participating, general surgery, 1990–1991

	Year	
	1990	1991
Surgeons contacted	1,025	1,004
Data returned	160	215
% Response	15.6	21.4

After collating and analysing the submissions, the surgeons are ranked according to their mortality and wound infection rates, etc, and each surgeon is informed in confidence of where he stands in that analysis, so that he can see his position in relation to the rest of the group. The resources available to him, the work-load which he or she undertakes, and other complications are also tabulated. Each year, two specific topics are analysed in more detail. Laparoscopic cholecystectomy was introduced into this country in 1990, so it was exciting to study the results of this new procedure in successive years. Other general surgical topics so far studied include colorectal resection and the results of surgery for aortic aneurysm.

The service has now expanded to include orthopaedic and ear, nose and throat surgeons. The urologists and paediatric surgeons are also joining, and several other surgical disciplines may take part later. Each discipline surveys two specific subtopics in addition to overall practice figures.

Cholecystectomy survey

As an example, I describe some of the results of our cholecystectomy survey, carried out in 1991–92. To date, details have been received on 7,755 open cholecystectomies and 2,427 laparoscopic cholecystectomies. Although 5% of the latter required conversion to an open operation, the complication rate after laparoscopic cholecystectomy (7.1%) was less than for open (13.1%), and the mortality rate (0.2%) was one-quarter of that of open cholecystectomy (0.8%). These are creditable results, bearing in mind that surgeons were developing new laparoscopic techniques during 1990 and 1991. Review of individual complication rates gives an example of what can be learnt by gathering these data.

Open cholecystectomies were found to be associated with a much higher complication rate in terms of systemic problems. A large abdominal incision increases the risk of chest infections, circulatory problems, urinary retention, etc, so the incidence of these is less with a smaller incision and a shorter hospital stay. However, the risk of damage to the bile ducts in laparoscopic cholecystectomy is slightly greater than with open surgery, although the difference is not statistically significant. The most important point for surgeons in doing laparoscopic gall bladder surgery is to avoid bile duct injury. Such findings illustrate the power of multicentre surgical audit using a common data set.

Reference

1. Campling EA, Devlin HB, Hoile RW, Lunn JN. *The Report of the National Confidential Enquiry into Perioperative Deaths 1991/2*. London: NCEPOD, Royal College of Surgeons, 1993

7 | Royal College of Obstetricians and Gynaecologists

Michael Maresh
Director, Medical Audit Unit, Royal College of Obstetricians and Gynaecologists

The Royal College of Obstetricians and Gynaecologists, unlike most other Colleges, used its core funding from the Department of Health to set up a medical audit unit based in a hospital, St Mary's Hospital for Women and Children, Manchester. This hospital is part of a large complex of hospitals, Central Manchester Health Care Trust, which is a major university hospital and a tertiary referral centre. Siting the unit in a hospital gives ready access to clinical material for developing audit.

The audit unit has three main functions:

- to provide a help desk and database on audit in obstetrics and gynaecology;
- to develop audit in more difficult areas; and
- to provide large-scale audit infrastructure.

Help desk and database on audit in obstetrics and gynaecology

Topics for audit, adverse events that might be monitored and effective protocols to use can be suggested to the many people who still find it difficult to start audit and also to clinicians and audit facilitators who have run out of ideas. Suitable topics to audit include the use of corticosteriods prior to pre-term delivery, suture techniques for the perineum, and case note completion. We also advise people to audit areas in which patient perspectives are prominent, a good example of which is threatened miscarriage, which occurs frequently.

The results of successful audit are distributed, and advice can be given on the standards which exist, as well as ensuring that only effective procedures are used. In obstetrics there is a useful data source.[1] (The authors also produce a regularly updated computerised database.[2])

Maternal deaths have been monitored since 1952, and an extensive national perinatal mortality enquiry is just beginning.

Of more value locally is the morbidity in obstetrics and gynaecology. Units can be advised to investigate all cases in which mature babies have to be admitted for neonatal special care (an indicator of intrapartum care) or all cases of undiagnosed congenital abnormalities (an indicator of antenatal management), and be advised on what levels of both might be expected. Suitable subjects for review with regard to maternal morbidity are cases of eclampsia, failed forceps deliveries and major genital tract trauma. Suitable topics for audit of gynaecological morbidity are various basic surgical outcomes and adverse events such as rates of blood tranfusion, re-admission and transfer to intensive care.

Busy clinicians often do not have the time to do the necessary background work for an audit, so it is helpful to have someone at the end of a telephone to give advice or who can send them some of the successful protocols. Clinicians can be provided with a set of questions to develop locally with their own audit department.

A region is a useful size for a specialty audit in obstetrics and gynaecology. The numbers are large enough, and the clinicians know one another. I recently surveyed all 68 gynaecologists in our region, all of whom responded. It would be difficult for either an individual audit facilitator or the regional audit lead to obtain a 100% response to a postal survey from clinicians. This illustrates the importance of leadership in audit coming from the top, from the College, as well as having consultant involvement.

A database has been developed which is seen as a central component of the unit. It contains the names of all lead audit clinicians and audit facilitators in the United Kingdom. When an audit protocol has been developed and shown to work successfully, it is stored on this database — so that audit activity is updated continually. The database information includes the use of computerised audit systems and a literature database is being built up.

Developing audit in more difficult areas

The medical audit unit is also actively involved in some of the more controversial and difficult areas of audit in obstetrics and gynaecology: for example, the rate of Caesarean section in women having their first baby. The literature can give general assistance, but a hospital needs to know whether a detailed audit of its Caesarean sections should be done or whether its rate is satisfactory and limited resources can be concentrated on other audits.

By looking at work in a number of hospitals, such as ours and those in the North-West Thames region, it has been possible to avoid the problems of case mix and to develop a threshold for Caesarean sections in a 'standard primapara' (a woman in her first pregnancy who has reached 37 weeks, who does not have twins and whose baby is not presenting by the breech). All hospitals can use this, irrespective of case mix, and they need carry out a detailed study only if this threshold figure is exceeded.

An important common problem to address in gynaecology is cervical intra–epithelial neoplasia, because there may be serious sequelae and patient perspectives and anxieties are prominent. Cervical cytology, colposcopy and treatment to the cervix are all areas suitable for audit. As a start, 100 cone biopsies of the cervix in our hospital were reviewed to develop a threshold for complete excision of the lesion. The results have been presented to colleagues in other hospitals in the North-West Region, and they are being encouraged to do the same type of review.

Another area is the move to clinical (interdisciplinary) audit. This is seen as an important function for the unit. An example is antenatal care of healthy women. This involves midwives and general practitioners who have a major role in looking after healthy women. Consultant obstetricians have less involvement unless something begins to go wrong. All involved need to develop and agree standards.

Large-scale audit infrastructure

The College's audit unit in Manchester also provides an infrastructure for large-scale audits. Three subjects are in varying stages of completion.

Eclampsia

The British eclampsia survey team (BEST) study was performed in 1992. Although not based in our unit, much of the funding came from our central funding from the Department of Health. It was an epidemiological study of all cases of eclampsia occurring in hospitals in the United Kingdom. Eclampsia and hypertensive disease remains the major cause of maternal mortality.

Data were extracted from case notes and from general practitioner questionnaires. Over 500 cases have been identified — almost certainly nearly all the cases because complicated methods were used to ensure that cases were not missed. The study has produced clear data on this large number of women with eclampsia and how they were managed, from which it will be possible to derive the incidence of eclampsia and its mortality. More importantly, these cases can be reviewed to elucidate the problems of clinical management, hope-fully leading to a further refinement of management protocols.

Pre-natal diagnosis

A second major audit is a pre-natal diagnosis study in eight hospi-tals across two regions. Both teaching and non-teaching units are being studied, and the audit investigates four areas:

- How good are we in practice at identifying risk factors for con-genital abnormalities in the antenatal period?
- Are appropriate tests being offered?
- Are women satisfied with the tests?
- Are women satisfied with their care when an abnormality is diagnosed?

The full study will be completed in mid-1993, but the prelimi-nary analysis shows that guidelines are not always clear enough and are often not applied in practice.

Minimally invasive techniques for treating menorrhagia

A confidential enquiry is being performed on the treatment of heavy menstrual bleeding (menorrhagia) using the new minimally invasive techniques, which are now being widely introduced as an alternative to hysterectomy. This study commenced in April 1993 and is scheduled to last for one year.

All cases of endometrial ablation and resection, and radiofre-quency ablation or cryoablation will be studied, whether performed in the health service or private sector. The study with the acronym 'MISTLETOE' (minimally invasive surgical techniques, laser endothermal or endoresection) will look at the frequency of use and of complications, and at the types of complications. It will be linked in confidence with the experience of surgeons. Hopefully, some standards can be developed in terms of who should do the procedures and what training they should be given. This study will also provide a large cohort of women who can be followed up for long-term studies.

Reference

1. Chalmers I, Kierse MJNC, Enkin M, eds. *Effective care in pregnancy and childbirth.* Oxford: Oxford University Press, 1989
2. The Cochrane Collaboration Pregnancy and Childbirth Database. Cochrane Centre, 1993

8 | Royal College of Pathologists

Gifford Batstone
Consultant Chemical Pathologist, Salisbury General Hospital

Pathology has a long tradition of a systematic, critical review of the quality of its services:

- with respect to analytical performance of pathology laboratories;
- by relating to the quality of patient care through the clinico-pathology conference;
- by leading cross-infection control and similar activities; and
- through working with clinical colleagues in agreeing guidelines for appropriate investigations.

These activities form the basis for the evolution of medical and clinical audit in pathology.

Performance of pathology laboratories

The external quality assessment schemes (EQAs) have been the mainstay of validation of the accuracy and precision of analytical results used by physicians, surgeons and general practitioners.[1] All pathology laboratories are expected to participate in an EQA scheme for the analyses they undertake where a suitable scheme exists, and nearly all laboratories do so at present. There are some 70 such schemes running nationally and locally which cover the activities undertaken in pathology departments, ranging from general chemistry for urea and electrolytes to specialist areas such as neuropathology. Increasingly, EQAs address not only technical performance but also the clinical interpretation of findings. Samples are sent 'blind' to participating laboratories, which are given a short time to analyse and interpret the findings before returning their results. Returns are collated, and the laboratories receive information on the distribution of results by participants, including as a subgroup those using their particular method and/or equipment. In this way, pathologists can both give assurance to users of their services about the quality of their work and also act in areas where performance is suboptimal. Those laboratories which consistently perform poorly are referred to a panel of experts who are able to help solve local problems. The criteria for acceptable performance are being uprated gradually as technological advances enable laboratories to gain greater precision of analysis.

Some laboratories are now turning this activity into an audit process by agreeing goals of analytical performance with users of their services. These then constitute the standards to be met. The results of EQAs are reviewed against these standards and action taken to maintain the quality of service at this agreed level.

The Royal College of Pathologists has been closely involved for the past three years, in instituting clinical pathology accreditation (CPA),[2] an important development which will give further assurance to users and purchasers of laboratory services that they are obtaining good quality. The CPA has set 44 criteria by which all aspects of a pathology department may be assessed under the six headings of personnel, facilities and equipment, policies, procedures, education, and quality assessment.[3] There is also a requirement to undertake clinical audit and to provide information to assist the audit of clinical colleagues.

Each laboratory interprets the criteria with the help of advice, and determines whether it meets those standards or should undertake necessary action to meet them. An inspection team of two people then visits each laboratory to determine whether or not they agree that these criteria of performance have been met. As an example, under the heading 'Facilities and equipment' is the statement: 'There is appropriate, properly maintained scientific equipment to meet the demands of the service' — followed by some explanatory comments. The laboratory staff review this measure and assess whether or not they are able to provide information that, for instance, they have standards for the maintenance of equipment together with evidence that such standards are met. If the laboratory is of the opinion that it has, it indicates this to the CPA. Soon after a laboratory has completed its own assessment of its performance against the 44 criteria, CPA sends two inspectors to provide a peer assessment. This includes not only a review of standards but also an interview with users of the service and general management. Based on the inspectors' report, CPA determines whether to grant accreditation. This process of accreditation allows laboratories to set standards against pre-determined criteria of laboratory practice, to assess their own performance and then undergo peer review. It therefore encompasses many of the elements of an audit process.

To date, CPA has received more than 850 requests for documentation and about 240 formal applications, and has given full accreditation to more than 80 laboratory departments. The pilot studies of this system revealed minor problems in about 40% of laboratories and major problems in almost 10%.[4] Participants in these pilot projects consider that substantial benefits of subjecting themselves to CPA inspection were apparent a year later.[5]

Another route to quality enhancement in areas of specialist interest has been through tumour registries, for example, of bone tumours, and clubs such as the Melanoma Club. Through circulation of histological material to members, these special interest groups are able to compare opinions with respect to problem cases and, with time, assess these opinions against the clinical history and survival of patients — thus completing an audit loop. For more routine histology, it is common practice for histologists to exchange one in fifteen slides with a colleague to promote discussion of ideas, keeping up-to-date with practice, and improving quality.

The clinico-pathology conference

Most hospitals have regular clinico-pathology meetings in which the findings and actions of clinical staff are related to the those of investigative departments, particularly the post-mortem findings. Through such enquiry, it is often possible to determine ways in which clinical practice may be improved — indeed, there is often an exhortation that practice should be different in future. However, the limitation of these meetings has frequently been failure to check that future practice *has* been enhanced. The introduction of such a check process converts these important meetings into audit by the process of 'closing the loop'. This is a significant extension to the current role of the clinico-pathology conference, but an important one for enhancing the quality of patient care.

Leading activities that enhance the quality of patient care

Microbiologists, usually working with cross-infection control nurses and a supporting committee, have an essential role in checking the sterility of hospital areas such as operating theatres, and in devising ward techniques which minimise the risk of infection. They also monitor patterns of infection to show possible cross-infection. Unfortunately, such activity is rarely linked with medical and clinical audit although, as with clinico-pathology conferences, it is the basis of good audit practice. A system of reporting findings to medical audit groups should enable the audit cycle to be completed and the work of these committees enhanced. Similar arguments may be made for other committees in which pathologists play major roles through their expert knowledge — antibiotic policy groups, blood products committees and so on.

Working with colleagues in agreeing guidelines for appropriate investigations

Pathologists have sought for many years to gain agreement with colleagues on information which would enhance the appropriate use of pathology services. Many laboratories have produced handbooks for new junior doctors and for general practitioners (as required for CPA), but more recently the focus has changed as more disease or condition-specific guidelines are produced which often cover both primary and secondary aspects of patient care. The pathologist has had a considerable role in the production of guidelines on care of diabetes, measurement of serum cholesterol and management of infections. These guidelines, like those produced by medical Royal Colleges and speciality groups, are rich source material for medical audit. Investigation guidelines prepared in Birmingham are now undergoing field trials in anticipation that they will become established markers of good practice and open to the scrutiny of audit.[6]

The nature of medical audit in pathology

Whilst the activities of pathologists listed above indicate a background of critical enquiry into the quality of patient care which may be extended to become medical and clinical audit, there are other audit processes in which the specialty is involved. Pathology has a strong influence on the success of some national audit projects, in particular, the National Confidential Enquiry into Perioperative Deaths (NCEPOD) and Confidential Enquiry into Stillbirths and Deaths in Infancy (CESDI).

The joint publication of the Colleges of Pathologists, Physicians and Surgeons entitled 'Autopsy and audit',[7] indicates the importance of post-mortem examinations in improving the quality of patient care. Associated with this approach are a number of interesting developments in audit in pathology such as criteria for EQA schemes, cervical cytology proficiency testing, and the quality of autopsy examinations.

The College has recently formed an audit committee charged with disseminating good audit practice and with promulgating new approaches and national audit projects.

A number of other audit techniques are being used in pathology. The EQA schemes have implicit standards insofar as it is considered that the median position within a group is the accepted standard of analysis and the basis consensus comparison. Detailed enquiry into sentinel events, such as a blood transfusion reaction, to ensure that guidelines have been followed, is another approach to audit. Cross-correlation with other diagnostic techniques such as diagnostic imaging forms an interesting approach to audit. For instance, histological findings from colectomy may be compared with those of colonoscopy and barium enema, or liver biopsy findings with ultrasound, biochemical and immunological data.

Increasingly, criterion-referenced medical audit is being undertaken. It is often convenient to view audit projects from the standpoints of access, process, outputs, outcomes and use of resources. In this context, accessibility of the service relates to collection of samples, readily available information on the right container for a specimen and tube volumes required, availability out-of-hours; process to accuracy and precision of results, timeliness and turn-around time; outputs relate to the usage by the clinical team. The measurement of outcomes assesses the benefit to patients derived from the investigations. The measurement of the use of resources links to resource management.

At a local level, pathologists' views of audit cover their three roles:

- the pathologist as a doctor: the quality of his or her clinical opinion on histological preparations or on data generated by analytical techniques. This concerns the pathologist's personal craft and knowledge;
- the pathologist as the leader of a multidisciplinary team: the way in which the department is run overall; and
- the role of the pathologist in assessing the effectiveness of laboratory services: this is a collaborative approach with clinical colleagues to determine whether or not appropriate use is made of laboratory services, and whether appropriate action is taken on the basis of results.

Another way to look at the activity of pathology laboratories is to divide activity into:

- pre-analytical, which deals with the range of tests available and whether or not requests match clinical need;
- analytical, which deals with the processes monitored by EQAs, but also reviews timeliness of responses; and
- post-analytical, which is concerned with the response of doctors to the pathology information provided at their request.

In conclusion the specialty of pathology has a long tradition in audit related activities such as the clinicopathological conference, infection control and the effective and appropriate use of laboratory facilities. This has changed from placing most emphasis on technical quality through quality assurance schemes and ways of gaining a more rapid response to requests to the current position where pathology is well placed to audit the pre and post analytical aspects of the pathologists work in collaboration with other medical specialties.

References

1. United Kingdom. National Quality Assurance Schemes, Report and Directory. Sheffield: NEQAS, 1993
2. The College Accreditation Steering Committee. Royal College of Pathologists' United Kingdom pilot study of laboratory accreditation. *Journal of Clinical Pathology* 1990; **43**: 89–91
3. The College Accreditation Steering Committee. Pathology department accreditation in the United Kingdom: a synopsis. *Journal of Clinical Pathology* 1991; **44**: 798–802
4. Report on the second study of laboratory accreditation. Sheffield: Clinical Pathology Accreditation, 1991
5. The College Accreditation Steering Committee. Royal College of Pathologists' accreditation pilot study: a year later. *Journal of Clinical Pathology* 1991; **44**: 172–3
6. Mutimer D, McCauley B, Nightingale P, *et al.* Computerised protocols for laboratory investigation and their effects on use of medical time and resources. *Journal of Clinical Pathology,* 1992; **45**: 572–4
7. Royal College of Pathologists, Royal College of Physicians and Royal College of Surgeons. *Autopsy and audit.* London: Royal College of Pathologists, 1990

9 | Royal College of Anaesthetists

Joseph Stoddart
Consultant in Charge, Intensive Therapy Unit,
Royal Victoria Infirmary, Newcastle upon Tyne

Anaesthetists have been involved in audit of their own activities for many years. An example of this was in 1956 when a report on 1,000 deaths associated with anaesthesia was published and its recommendations widely followed.[1] Later development in anaesthetic audit led to the establishment of the National Confidential Enquiry into Perioperative Deaths (NCEPOD) which has become the standard with which many such activities are compared.[2]

The Royal College of Anaesthetist's audit committee was renamed the Quality of Practice Committee in 1989 to emphasise that its ultimate objective is to improve standards of care. The membership of the committee includes six members of the Council of the College, with representatives from NCEPOD, the Intensive Care Society, the Pain Society, the Association of Anaesthetists, and the Department of Health. The committee's objectives are to initiate, assess and support audit activities proposed by Fellows of the College. It was initially funded by the College, but now receives most of its funding from the Department of Health, with some support from the Welsh Office and the Northern Ireland Health Department.

The College has stated in its guidelines that participation in audit on a regular and recorded basis is a mandatory requirement for recognition of the hospital for the training of junior staff. The educational aspect of audit is widely appreciated. The College has introduced a log-book for trainees. This includes a minimum data set about training, but in addition allows the College visitor to discuss with the trainee gaps and needs in the training programme, and also to discern whether or not the trainee is being correctly supervised.

Anaesthetists are particularly concerned at the relatively poor standard of anaesthetic record keeping and the low priority attached to it by hospital records' departments — a concern that has both clinical and medico-legal implications. The College is looking into methods of automatic and semi-automatic computerised record keeping.

Audit and anonymity

A number of consultants have expressed anxiety about the accessibility of records of audit activities to the patient's legal representatives — and indeed to the patient himself. Many of the Colleges have sought legal advice on this matter. Anaesthetists have been told by their College that patients are interested only in their own records. Since these should be kept accurately and legibly, and are freely accessible to the patient or his representative, no additional liability is generated by collation of such data either regionally or centrally. If and when some adverse outcome occurs, this should of course be correctly recorded. It is equally important to state that any identified cause should be noted but not commented upon.

It is both unprofessional and unwise to make adverse comments which may attribute blame, either in public, for example at audit meetings, or in print on a patient's records. In particular, junior staff must not be criticised at audit meetings or they will decline to take part.

Past and current activities

The Quality of Practice committee invites applications for audit grants. The applications are subject to expert scrutiny before decisions are taken concerning their support. Funds are provided for a wide variety of purposes, including salaries, equipment and general expenses. A number of projects have recently been completed. These include:

- a pilot study on the value of critical incident monitoring — this is particularly important since anaesthesia is regarded by the legal profession as a 'dangerous' speciality which is subject to litigation;
- a survey of the incidence of unexpected cardiac arrest and brain damage associated with surgery and anaesthesia;
- a review of the type of audit activities carried out in anaesthetic departments; and
- the neurological complications of obstetric epidural anaesthesia.

The Quality of Practice Committee is currently supporting two audit programmes (one of which is nationwide)[3] concerning the use of intensive therapy units and their activities. It has also given its support to a study of the need for, and availability of, pain relief in childhood, and has recently agreed to support an attempt to define factors which predict the course and outcome of cardiac surgery. The Committee also supports a separate regional study of outcome from cardiac surgery using a categorical multiple regression model.

Representatives of the committee are assisting in the compilation of a vocabulary of terms to permit Read coding of anaesthetic and intensive therapy unit activities.

Audit and the employing authority

Managers have a legitimate interest in certain aspects of audit, including the appropriate use of clinical time, operating theatre usage, bed occupancy in the intensive therapy unit and so on. The White Paper, *Working for Patients*,[4] clearly states that audit activities are regarded as mandatory and part of every doctor's clinical duty, and also spells out that there will be a recognised cost of this type of activity. The Royal College of Anaesthetists has stated that the practice of holding half-day audit meetings at monthly intervals on a rolling basis (ie Monday one month, Tuesday the next, etc.) has much to recommend it. In many hospitals this practice is being followed by all specialties simultaneously, so that shared audit activities can occur.

References

1. Edwards G, Morton HJV, Pask EA, Wylie WD. Deaths associated with anaesthesia: a report on 1000 cases. *Anaesthesia* 1956; **11**: 194–220
2. Campling EA, Devlin HB, Hoile RW, Lunn JN. *The Report of the National Confidential Enquiry into Perioperative Deaths 1991/2.* London: NCEPOD Royal College of Surgeons, 1993
3. National ITU Audit 1992/93. London: Royal College of Anaesthetists, 1993
4. Department of Health. *Working for Patients.* London: HMSO, 1989

10 | Royal College of Radiologists

Raymond Godwin
Chairman, Royal College of Radiologists Audit Working Party

Activity in the field of audit by the Royal College of Radiologists did not begin with the White Paper, *Working for patients,*[1] but preceded it with some early hard work in the mid-1970s. The College set up a working party in 1976 to look into ways of improving the use of radiological services nationally. Initially, a series of national multicentre studies was established to identify credible guidelines for a number of common X-ray examinations, including skull and pre-operative chest X-rays.

The first edition of the now well-known guidelines[2] was published in 1990, and promoted and distributed through the College audit office set up in 1991. More than 40,000 copies have been distributed widely throughout the health service to date, and many hospitals have accepted this document as their basis for guidance in radiology practice. The first edition contained 12 categories of X-ray procedure covering 70 important clinical circumstances, which together comprise 95% of all radiological investigations. As with all true audit processes, the effect of instituting these guidelines has been assessed in the setting of both hospital and general practice medicine. Two publications have identified that the effect of implementing the guidelines is typically a 20–25% reduction in requested examinations.[3,4]

Another paper on the effect of the guidelines on general practice has recently been published.[5] The second edition is now available, which includes guidance on the use of computerised tomographic scanning, ultrasound, nuclear medicine and mammography, greatly expanding its usefulness.[6] Guidance on the implementation of these guidelines has also been made available to Fellows of the College.

The audit office within the College functions for both the Faculties (Radiology and Clinical Oncology). It is an essential centre for the dissemination of audit information, facilitation of audit activities, and collection of audit information and local audit results. This last function is, however, slow to develop. A national database of radiologists with local audit responsibility is held by the office, thus simplifying the distribution of audit information.

Current activities

Radiology

A national audit of ilio-femoral angioplasty is currently under way. To date, more than 5,200 procedures have been recorded. After a two-year period of patient follow-up, standards should be identifiable against which individual departments can audit their own activity in and results of this procedure using nationally available figures. Other audits of interventional radiological procedures are likely to be based upon this initial study. Discussions are currently taking place on a national audit of obstetric ultrasound in the district hospital setting.

Clinical Oncology

In 1989, Priestman *et al.* published a paper showing a wide variation in the dose/fraction regimen in the treatment of common conditions requiring radiotherapy.[7] Training and established local policies emerged as major influences on practice, with only a small effect from clinical trials. A case was made for further national studies under the auspices of the Royal College of Radiologists, with financial support from the Department of Health, with the aim of making recommendations for the best treatment regimen.

The first of these studies was carried out in non-small-cell lung cancer,[8] which accounts for 10–20% of the workload in departments of radiotherapy. All 54 radiotherapy units in the United Kingdom have been involved in it.

The second study to develop guidelines for treatment will be on early breast cancer and will be under the aegis of the Joint Council for Clinical Oncology, which includes representatives of the Royal Colleges of Radiologists and Physicians.

Work on reducing delays in cancer treatment is also in progress, with the setting of treatment targets to improve services. These standards and targets will need to be nationally audited if improvement in services is to be encouraged, a process which the College is ideally placed to perform.

A further proposed project is the clinical oncology information network (COIN), under the leadership of Dr Stephen Karp. This is a clinical information system suitable for use by all cancer centres. The use of such a common system of information gathering would enable a national comparative audit to be facilitated and a national clinical oncology database created.

In response to the joint publication of the Royal College of Radiologists and the National Radiation Protection Board, *Reducing patient dosage*,[9] a nationwide audit is currently being organised by the College to discover what has been the response to the 22 recommendations in this publication.

Education in audit, and the assurance that audit is being used in education and as a guide to educational needs, remain a primary function of the college. About 14 months ago a survey of College Members and Fellows showed that 96% of them were carrying out audit. This was a pleasing reponse, but 76% of them also said that in fact they knew little or nothing about audit. It is hoped that this situation has now improved.

Continuing medical education, including audit, is uppermost in the College's plans for the future. There is a lack of funding in some hospitals for consultant study leave. Audit can identify educational need effectively and also help to justify the funding allocation for it.

The development of national standards applicable to radiology departments leads to the possibility of a form of departmental accreditation. These ideas are currently being developed, and some form of accreditation is under consideration by the College.

References

1.   Department of Health. *Working for patients.* London: HMSO, 1989
2.   Royal College of Radiologists. *Making the best use of a department of radiology. Guidelines for doctors.* London: Royal College of Radiologists. 1990
3.   A multicentre audit of hospital referral for radiological investigation in England and Wales. *British Medical Journal* 1991; **303**: 809–12
4.   Royal College of Radiologists. Influence of the Royal College of Radiologists' guidelines on hospital practice: a multicentre study. Britsh Medical Journal 1992; **304**: 740–743
5.   Royal College of Radiologists. Influence of the Royal College of Radiologists' guidelines on referral from general practice. *British Medical Journal* 1993; **306**: 110–1
6.   Royal College of Radiologists. *Making the best use of a department of clinical radiology — guidelines for doctors.* Second edition; London: Royal College of Radiologists, 1993
7.   Priestman TJ, Bullimore JA, Godden TP, Deutsch GP. The Royal College of Radiologists' Fractionation Survey. *Clinical Oncology* 1989; 1:39–46
8.   Maher EJ, Timothy A, Squire CJ, Goodman A, Karp SJ, Paine CH, Ryall R, Read G. Audit: the use of radiotherapy for non-small cell lung cancer in the UK. *Clinical Oncology* 1993; **5**: 72–79

9. Royal College of Radiologists and National Radiation Protection
    Board. *Patient dose reduction in diagnostic radiology.* National Radiation
    Protection Board vol 1, number 3. London: HMSO, 1990

11 | Royal College of Ophthalmologists

Brian Martin
Consultant Ophthalmic Surgeon, General Infirmary at Leeds

The audit unit of the Royal College of Ophthalmologists was formed in 1990. It is situated at the College, and is run by an audit committee. The committee consists of six consultant ophthalmologists, a representative from the Department of Health and an audit research fellow who was appointed in 1990 for a three-year period.

The audit group plans to collect data that are both valid and representative of current practice in ophthalmology, so that the inferences drawn from the results may be used by the College to influence health policy and the provision of ophthalmic services in the United Kingdom. The data will be used to develop practice guidelines that are practical and attainable, while being acceptable and workable by our colleagues.

To date, the College has undertaken the major part of the audit projects that have been set up, and the protocols and proformas have been written by the audit committee. Questionnaires have originated from the College unit, and the data have been collected at the College, where the projects have also been written up and submitted for publication.

Cataract

Cataract is one of the major causes of visual loss in the United Kingdom, and is the most eminently treatable. Cataract operations account for 60–70% of all major eye operations carried out in this country. A national cataract survey was designed to determine current surgical activity in relation to the delivery of the surgical service and the outcome of the surgical procedure. A prospective cross-sectional survey was carried out in week 48 of 1990. All consultant ophthalmologists in the United Kingdom were invited to participate, and were sent a proforma asking them to include all adult patients admitted for surgery for age-related cataract during the survey week. Patients having a combined procedure, for example, surgery for glaucoma and cataract, or who might have, for example, traumatic or congenital cataract, were excluded from the study.

The response was rather disappointing compared to that achieved in some other audit projects, for only 60% of eligible consultants replied. However, there was representation from 85% of all ophthalmic units in the United Kingdom, and all regions were represented. Almost 1,500 patients were included in the survey, 919 female and 575 male, with a mean age of 75.9 years.

In the last ten years there has been a move from intracapsular cataract surgery to the extracapsular method, with 92% of all procedures done by the latter method. Phakoemulsification is a relatively new method of removing cataracts. This technique allows a much smaller incision to be made into the eye, a much more rapid visual rehabilitation of the patient, and an even shorter stay in hospital. It also facilitates day-case surgery, but only 4% of operations were carried out in this way. The technique has yet to become universally accepted, and the equipment is not available in all ophthalmic units. Only 8% of all the cataract operations by whatever method carried out in this survey were performed as day cases — well below the Audit Commission's aim that 20% of cataract operations will ultimately be performed as day surgery.

The arguments for day-case surgery in ophthalmology are somewhat different to those in other specialties. The limit on the number of cataract operations performed is not due to a shortage of beds as, for example, in general surgery, but to a lack of surgical time. It is unlikely, therefore, that day-case surgery will increase throughput unless increased surgical time is provided either by an increase in the number of ophthalmologists or in the number of operating lists made available. It is, however possible, that there may be financial savings in day-case surgery. This audit project did not attempt to identify the outcomes of day-case surgery in contrast to inpatient surgery — a topic which should be audited in the future. Although over 40% of patients included in the survey had some form of co-existing ocular pathology, the results of cataract surgery were successful with 80% of patients achieving a visual acuity of between 6/6 and 6/12. Poor visual results were almost entirely due to pre-existing ocular pathology, seldom to any form of surgical or post-operative complication.

Ophthalmology is one of the specialties with long waiting lists, with many people waiting for cataract surgery for up to two years in some areas of the country. In this survey over 50% of patients had their operation within six months of being placed on the waiting list, although 17% waited more than one year.

An outcome study of cataract surgery concentrating on patient satisfaction will shortly commence in North-West Thames, involving three hospitals (a teaching hospital, an outer London Hospital, and one outside London). An attempt will be made to determine how much a patient's quality of life has been improved by this operation and whether or not an elderly patient benefits from surgery to the second eye.

Ocular trauma

The College is carrying out a further audit project designed to determine the causes, types and severity of ocular trauma in Scotland. Following the introduction of the requirement to wear seat belts in motor vehicles, penetrating ocular trauma has become much less common, but there are still considerable numbers of eye injuries requiring admission to hospital. This study is designed to give epidemiological information on this topic, to determine the outcome of treatment, and to enable the College to issue guidelines on the clinical assessment and management of such cases.

The other three principal causes of visual loss in the United Kingdom (diabetic retinopathy, glaucoma and age-related macular degeneration) are areas which the College plans to audit in the near future. It is probable that these projects will be carried out in a different manner to that previously used, for there is considerable benefit in devolving such audits to major centres away from the College and the audit unit. This will disseminate knowledge about audit. Planning and taking part in such audits are important educational exercises.

12 | Royal College of Physicians of London

Anthony Hopkins
Research Unit, Royal College of Physicians of London

The Royal College of Physicians of London has a number of initiatives in clinical audit. First, guidelines for good practice are being developed, almost always in association with the relevant specialist society. (A full list of those guidelines published and under development is available.[1])

Secondly, protocols for audit are being produced — that is, proformas which can be taken 'off the shelf' and used in different hospitals without further work. Before they are released for general consumption these protocols are usually piloted in a number of units to see whether they actually work and that the audit questions are not ambiguous. Protocols so far developed relate to the care of the elderly, stroke, diabetes mellitus, asthma and epilepsy. Others are at an advanced stage of preparation. However, I am bound to say that there is less enthusiasm for trying out the audit protocols than there is for developing the guidelines on which they are based.

The feasibility of routine diabetes audit is being tested out in four health districts, led by Philip Home in Newcastle. Asthma has been audited twice by an energetic group of respiratory physicians, after publication of guidelines developed jointly with the British Thoracic Society and the National Asthma Campaign.[2,3] Although respiratory physicians agreed the guidelines that were disseminated nationally, an audit one year after publication showed that practice was continuing much as before. Further research is needed into how physicians' practices can be changed. Is education enough, or are there other incentives that might have to be provided? Barbara Stocking considers the evidence for different methods of achieving change in chapter 21.

Nearly 90% of patients in medical beds have been admitted acutely, so acute medical admissions and outpatients together represent most of the work of physicians, the organisation of both of which aspects is often rather a muddle. Dr Anita Houghton and I have developed an audit protocol, and piloted it in eight hospitals, which explores how a hospital manages its acute admissions.[4] In this project we are not concerned with individual diseases, such as the management of myocardial infarction, upper gastro-intestinal haemorrhage and so on, but about the *organisation* of care. The protocol contains some interesting questions: for example, the switchboard supervisor is asked if he or she knows which physician and senior house officer are on duty that day.

For outpatients, the College has been developing a protocol with colleagues at St Mary's Hospital and with general practitioners in Parkside District. It is true to say that although a lot of effort has been put into this project, the audit system is not yet right. Perhaps it is over-ambitious, but an attempt is being made to go beyond waiting times and other administrative aspects of outpatients, which are easy enough to audit. Although these are important, they do not really inform us of the *clinical* quality of the outpatient service, which continues to be a major priority.

Another audit initiative relates to the perspectives of the users of health services. An audit protocol was developed, together with the Prince of Wales Advisory Trust, to explore the difficulties encountered in hospital by people with physical disabilities.[5] The Prince of Wales wrote a foreword to the protocol. Funds are now being sought to support disabled people so that they may audit their own local hospitals.

As another example of exploring the perspectives of users, the care given to people with brain tumours is being examined. Malignant gliomas have a grave prognosis. In terms of one measure of quality of life, the quality-adjusted life year (QALY), one publication suggests that their treatment is amongst the least efficient of medical technologies — £68,674 at 1984 prices per QALY.[6] My colleagues, Dr Charles Clarke and Dr Elizabeth Davies, and I have organised some focused interviews of patients and their spouses to try to find out what they think about their illness and its management. Is the best being done for such patients? Early results will be available in 1994.

To develop further these ideas about the perspectives of users of health services, two small books have been published on the measurement of the quality of life[7] and on the measurement of patient satisfaction.[8] I am keen always to stress the importance of measurement. Unless an aspect of health care or outcome can be measured, it is hardly worth talking about.

Finally, two health service research projects: the first, again with Dr Houghton, and supported by the Wellcome Trust, is to explore whether a discharge planner, a person paid specifically to do this job, is more effective than leaving the task to the ward sisters and

house physicians. The second, with Dr Zarrina Kurtz, and supported by College Appeal Funds and South-West Thames Regional
Health Authority, is an exploration of the systems needed to
ensure that children growing up with chronic disorders like cystic
fibrosis or epilepsy are moved into systems of care and support
appropriate for adult life, and are not abandoned at the point of
transition between childhood and adult life.

One future initiative will relate to outcomes research. How can
specialist colleagues define the outcomes of their interventions? A
necessary subsidiary question is how can raw measures of outcome
be corrected for differences in severity of illness and comorbidity?
As recent newspaper headlines and correspondence have made
clear, outcomes between health regions or hospital units cannot
begin to be compared without correcting for case mix. Items other
than technical measures of case severity need to be taken into
account. For example, a woman stroke patient may be in hospital
for the good reason that her husband has just broken his hip, and
she cannot be sent home because there is nobody to look after her.
Unless that data item is recorded, the admission or day of care may
appear to be an inappropriate admission. There are enormous
complexities about clinical information which are only just beginning to be understood, and which the Clinical Terms Project
(Chapter 13) is only just beginning to unravel.

We are also considering how the college can best help purchasers. The guidelines so far prepared (eg Refs 8, 9) relate to professional and technical aspects of medical practice. How can these
be made accessible to purchasers, so that they can write contracts
specifying aspects of care that can be monitored?

References

1. Conference of Medical Royal Colleges and their Faculties in the UK.
   *Clinical audit activities of the Medical Royal Colleges and their Faculties in
   the United Kingdom.* London: Conference of Colleges, 1994
2. Statement by the British Thoracic Society, Research Unit of the Royal
   College of Physicians of London, King's Fund Centre, National Asthma Campaign. Guidelines for management of asthma in adults: I —
   acute severe asthma. *British Medical Journal* 1990; **301**: 651–3
3. British Thoracic Society, British Paediatric Association, Research Unit
   of the Royal College of Physicians of London, King's Fund Centre,
   National Asthma Campaign, Royal College of General Practitioners,
   General Practitioners in Asthma Group, British Association of
   Accident and Emerency Medicine, British Paediatric Respiratory
   Group, Guidelines on the management of asthma. *Thorax* 1993: **48**:
   S1–S24

4. Houghton A, Hopkins A. The development of an audit protocol for acute medical admissions. *Quality in Health Care* (in press)
5. A charter for disabled people using hospitals. London: Royal College of Physicians and the Prince of Wales Advisory Trust, 1992
6. Pickard JD, Bailey S, Sanderson H, Rees M, Garfield J. Steps towards cost-benefit analysis of regional neurosurgical care. *British Medical Journal* 1990; **301**: 629–35
7. Hopkins A, ed. *Measures of the quality of life — and the uses to which they may be put.* London: RCP Publications, 1992
8. Hopkins A, Fitzpatrick R, eds. *Measurement of patients' satisfaction with their care.* London: RCP Publications, 1993
9. Report of a working group of the Research Unit, Royal College of Physicians. Guidelines for the management of urinary infections in childhood. *Journal of the Royal College of Physicians of London* 1991; **25**: 36–42
10. de Bono D, Hopkins A. The investigation and management of stable angina. *Journal of the Royal College of Physicians of London* 1993; **27**: 267–73

DISCUSSION

Charles Shaw: Many of the Colleges are running national clinical audit studies. Much attention goes into designing the collection of data and writing reports, but I do not believe sufficient attention is paid to how the results of audit will be implemented locally. I suggest that the publication of the results of every national audit study should be associated with some advice about local audit.

Anthony Hopkins: This is where purchasers should come in. They could require in any contract either that the results (in broad terms) of any audit are made available to them, or that a provider unit takes part in a relevant national audit, for example, the confidential comparative audit of the Royal College of Surgeons.

Robert Johnson: A great deal has been heard about the development of clinical audit, and there is a lot of enthusiasm for good practice. Most of the 200 consultants in my hospital take part in audit, but a small number of doctors neither contribute to audit nor attend audit meetings. What are the views on 'policing' and enforcing audit? How should we act towards those consultants who do not contribute?

David Dunn: In future, purchasers may not place contracts with providers who cannot convince them that they are taking part in good audits and achieving good results. Such policies would surely influence all consultants: if they do not respond, they will not win contracts in the future.

Gifford Batstone: Clinical pathology accreditation is a purely professional matter, but it is also a marker for purchasers of the quality of the laboratory. Accreditation requires that all pathologists audit their own activity and join in the audit activities of others.

Joseph Stoddart: The Royal College of Anaesthetists is considering the use of a system of credits in which consultants have certain tasks which they need to fulfil each year. These include attendances at, and recognised contributions to meetings, and so on. They will keep a log-book of their activities which will be assessed by the College at periodic intervals to see whether consultants who have junior doctors working with them deserve their continuing status as teachers.

James Millar: Could the Chairman of the Conference of Colleges, give us some authoritative guidance on the question of protected time which should be made available to doctors working in hospital both for medical audit and for post-graduate education? In some cases, time for audit has come out of the limited time already available for post-graduate education.

Sir Stanley Simmons: The Colleges, Conference and Joint Consultants Committee are well aware of the pressures on consultants, and continue to draw this to the attention of the Department of Health and Ministers. Conference has declared that, on average, each doctor should spend 5% of his or her time on audit activities which, in a ten-session week, forty-session month, means one session every two weeks.

Section 3

Information management, information technology and clinical audit

13 | The Clinical Terms Project

James Read
Director, National Health Service Centre for Coding and Classification

---

The Clinical Terms Project was launched in April 1992. It is a collaborative project between the medical profession and the Information Management Group of the National Health Service (NHS) Management Executive to develop an agreed thesaurus of clinical terms sufficiently comprehensive to express anything a clinician might need to enter in a patient's record. The development of this dictionary of clinical terms is one of the main initiatives in the NHS Management and Technology Strategy,[1] and is being co-ordinated by the NHS Centre for Coding and Classification, a branch of the Information Management Group.

Patient-centred information system

Recent years have seen a significant change in the approach to information systems, with a shift in focus from simply collecting data and central returns for management purposes to patient–centred systems to support individual care (Figure 1). If the information collected is to be accurate and timely, it is important to involve the clinician. Patient-centred information systems have to be designed to make data entry and retrieval easy and, most importantly, to help clinicians look after patients. This patient-clinician interface is fundamental. The capture and use of data at the point of contact with the patient have to be as easy as writing in the clinical record — otherwise clinicians will not use the system. This vital issue is being addressed by a closely linked project, the Integrated Clinical Workstation Project, the aim of which is to produce a detailed specification of the requirements of clinical users. Several prototype demonstrators are planned in order to show how information required by practitioners may be collected and used in an integrated way.

It is a cardinal principle that information collected about individual patients should be entered only once and near to the patient, and also that data should be standard, transferrable and accessible wherever a patient is seen. The clinical data will then act

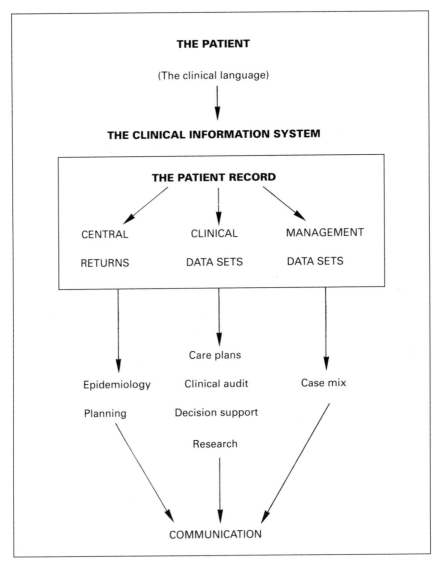

Fig 1. *The clinical information system.*

as a focal point to satisfy the data requirements for care plans, audit, protocols, decision support, and research. Systems should collect data that will help clinicians care for patients. Those same data can be used, as a by-product, throughout the NHS for local and central management purposes.

A language for health — The Clinical Terms Project

In 1991, a joint working group was set up consisting of

representatives of the Conference of Medical Royal Colleges and
their Faculties in the United Kingdom (the Conference), the Joint
Consultants Committee, the General Medical Services Committee
of the British Medical Association, and the NHS Management
Executive. Its purpose was to advise the NHS Chief Executive
about the information needs of clinicians and to ensure that, as far
as possible, NHS information strategy would be useful for patients.
At its first meeting, the group recognised that it was vital to establish an agreed dictionary (or thesaurus) of clinical terms, without
which information systems in the NHS could not store, compare
and transfer data. It was also agreed that the profession had to take
the lead in this project to ensure professional 'ownership'. The
Read codes had already been adopted as the standard clinical coding system for general practice,[5] and it was decided that they
should be adopted and expanded in all the various specialties to
enable them to be used throughout health care. The plan is to
agree a clinical thesaurus and to incorporate it into the Read
codes in a format suitable for use in the NHS information systems
by 1 April 1994.

Collecting a thesaurus of terms that clinicians write in their
records is only the first part of a major programme the objective of
which is to develop a full language for health. Having identified
the terms and allocated them codes within the Clinical Terms Project, these will then provide the building blocks on which other
work can build. This will include the definition of terms, their
incorporation into minimum data sets, classifications and groupings. The profession may then wish to assess their use in audit,
outcome measurement, research, and care plans.

This ability to capture and communicate information is central to
the new NHS Information Management and Technology strategy.[2] It
will be facilitated by developing the following components:

- a new format NHS number;
- shared NHS administrative registers;
- a national thesaurus of coded clinical terms;
- a system of NHS-wide networking;
- national standards for computer-to-computer communication;
  and
- a framework for security and confidentiality.

The development of a nationally agreed thesaurus of coded clinical terms is essential because useful communication is impossible
without a common language.[3] The thesaurus will also enable the
capture on computer of the individual patient record in far greater

detail than currently possible, including details of symptoms, signs, diagnosis, relevant procedures, therapies, pharmacological treatments, comorbidities, outcomes, social factors, and so on.

The Clinical Terms Project is thus simply about identifying the words and terms used to describe concepts that a clinician might need to write in a patient's record. It will define a preferred term for each concept and agree legitimate synonyms and eponyms, and other ways of describing these terms. These terms will then be allocated codes and cross-referenced or mapped to other recognised coding systems such as the International Classification of Diseases, 10th revision (ICD-10),[4] and will need to be arranged in an agreed structure to facilitate convenient search and display. Software requirements also have to be stipulated to make them usable.

A subset of the work has been to agree and define a list of clinical abbreviations by 1 April 1993. A defined list of acronyms will also be produced, the purpose of which is to identify those in common usage which would be used as 'keys' to facilitate the choice of terms for data entry. The working group also helped to pilot the organisation by the project of the collection and amalgamation of work from 40 specialty working groups. To date, almost 10,000 acronyms and abbreviations have been collected from the first 30 working groups which have returned them.

The NHS Centre for Coding and Classification is managing the project using the UK government standard project management methodology, PRojects IN Controlled Environments (PRINCE),[6] (Figure 2).

The members of the working groups have been selected by the profession. Each group consists of approximately seven senior clinical members, an appointed chairman and an associated research worker. Currently, there are 700 senior clinicians, including 70 professors, involved in the working groups.

Overall quality review for the project is provided by the project assurance team which mirrors the function of the project board by having members representing the business, technical and medical professions. The work of each working group is also reviewed by a speciality assurance team of three independent clinicians: an academic and an NHS consultant both from that specialty, and a general practitioner with an interest in it. Part of their responsibility is to ensure that the terms produced satisfy the detailed needs of the specialist, but also cater for the more general terminology required by other health care workers.

The chairmen of the specialty working groups, the project team and the Conference information group meet regularly at a user

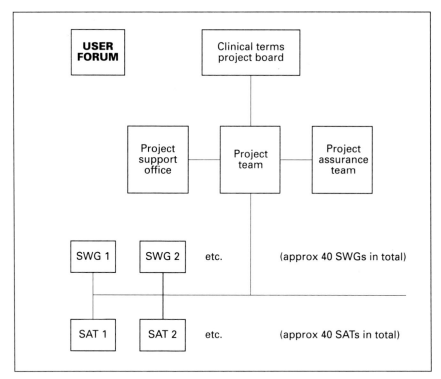

Fig 2. *The organisational structure of the Clinical Terms Project* (SWG: specialty working group; SAT: specialty assurance team).

forum to discuss ideas and issues arising during the progress of the project. During these forums, the needs for generic working groups are identified to tackle issues of terminology which cross specialties. These bring together key people from different working groups and other specialists to ensure a consistent and co-ordinated approach to a number of common concepts and key issues that most groups will need to address, such as care plans, outcome terms, complications of operations, symptomatology and other features of the patient encounter.

Similar projects have been established both for the nursing profession (nurses, midwives and health visitors) and for the professions allied to medicine (physiotherapy, occupational therapy, chiropody, dietetics, and speech and language therapy). These groups are increasingly contributing to almost all the medical specialty working groups, and the user forum now encompasses all these professions. This collaboration should ensure that the terms produced apply across professional boundaries, creating a truly shared language of health, for use by all health care workers for the benefit of patient care.

References

1. McSean T. NHS launches information strategy. *British Medical Journal* 1993; **306**:10
2. Information Management Group. *Information Management and Technology strategy overview.* Leeds: National Health Service Management Executive, 1992
3. Buckland R. The language of health. *British Medical Journal* 1993; **306**: 287-8
4. World Health Organisation. *International Classification of Diseases and Health related Behaviour.* Geneva: WHO, 1992
5. Chisholm J. The Read clinical classification. *British Medical Journal* 1990; **300**: 1092
6. Central Computing and Telecommunications Agency (CCTA). *The PRINCE* Reference manuals 1–5. Manchester: National Computing Centre Blackwell, 1990

14 | Links between resource management and clinical audit

Bob Broughton

Welsh Secretary, British Medical Association, formerly Adviser on Medical Audit, Welsh Health Common Services Authority

Over the last decade there has been a plethora of organisations, reorganisations, and initiatives in the National Health Service (NHS). Following the introduction of resource management, defined as a new initiative to involve health professionals in the management of NHS services and resources, there have been all the now familiar papers and strategies referring to items such as purchasing and providing, the formation of NHS trusts, the initiation of clinical audit and related quality issues, including total quality management, and of course both in England and Wales the publication of strategies for health care (described in Wales as a series of protocols for health gain). If the medical profession could perceive the links between all these initiatives, and if these links could be identified as one unifying driving force that gathers together all the different strands, their understanding by clinicians would become much easier, and their implementation facilitated.

Managing doctors and their activities has been described as parallel to herding cats, so it is essential that the 'cats' should all perceive the need to go in the same direction. There is also an essential need for good clinical decision making to be founded on a degree of feline independence, so we may conclude that it is better to find common ground for the above-mentioned initiatives that encompass the clinical decision making process, rather than trying to constrain clinical decision making into pre-determined pathways. It is my belief that the pathways that link initiatives may be identified as the pathways down which data and information flow in the day-to-day organisation of health care. The strategy for information technology in Wales embraces the concept of installing operational systems that collect clinical and management information as a by-product of their operational purpose. The detail of these operational systems are being spelled out in the Welsh Clinical Management System Specification. This specification is currently

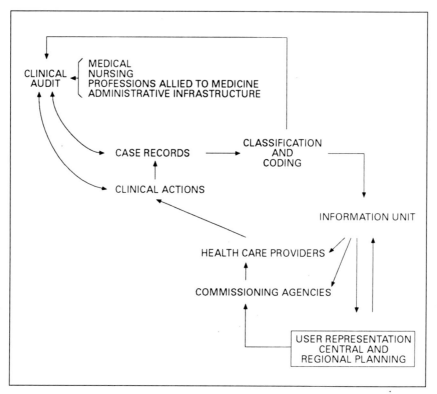

Fig 1. *Information pathways.*

being produced by the profession, and it links with other systems relating to associated health care professionals. It is then possible to identify the pathways down which the data so collected flow, linking up all the new initiatives, and all the different health care professionals involved in them, at the same time providing a unifying purpose and breaking down the compartments within the health service.

The data originate at the clinician-patient interface and are mostly recorded within the case record. They are then aggregated and processed for a variety of purposes, including clinical or professional audit. Data are also aggregated within the medical records department to provide statistics for management as well as for professional purposes, and are then processed via some coding or classification system for transmission to higher tiers of management. At each level the information becomes more aggregated and more sophisticated, but it can then be called back down to the operational level for purposes of planning and organisation.

These pathways have existed in Wales since the inception of the

NHS but the participants have changed. In the early days, the material was collected by the matron or a hospital secretary and aggregated in reports to boards of governors or to the Welsh Hospital Board. Over the years, the matron has become the director of nursing services or a chief administrative nursing officer, the hospital secretary a unit, sector, district or area administrator — and so forth — but the underlying pathways have remained intact. The scheme (shown in Figure 1) identifies these pathways in the context of the latest reforms, recognising the purchaser-provider split, the audit function, and the role of public health medicine both in monitoring the provision of health care and also in advising the purchaser on health needs assessment, in conjunction with central planning authorities.

15 | Confidentiality and clinical audit

John Wall
Chief Executive, The Medical Defence Union

Following the first report of the Confidential Enquiry into Perioperative Deaths (CEPOD)[1] and the White Paper, *Working for Patients*[2], which stated that:

> every consultant should participate in a form of medical audit agreed between management and the profession locally

— the Royal Colleges, British Medical Association and defence and protection societies, among others, have joined forces to discuss confidentiality in relation to medical audit. The Royal College of Surgeons in *Guidelines to clinical audit in surgical practice*[3] considered that 'confidentiality to the group is absolute'.

Working for Patients put a rather different emphasis:

> Peer review findings in individual cases should be confidential, but the general results of medical audit should be available to management locally and the lessons published more widely.

There is widespread public mistrust of 'confidential internal enquiries' into mishaps, but such enquiries do not define audit.

In a well-known case addressing the liability of relatively inexperienced junior hospital doctors, Vice-Chancellor Browne-Wilkinson (Wilsher v Essex Area Health Authority) said that a health authority:

> which so conducts its hospital that it fails to provide doctors of sufficient skill and experience to give the treatment offered at the hospital may be directly liable in negligence to the patient ... I can see no reason why, in principle, the health authority should not be so liable if its organisation is at fault.[4]

Therefore, if a trust hospital or directly managed unit in an attempt to assess risk, including the risk of inadequate experience on the part of the doctors who staff its wards and clinics, insists on a quality assurance programme but does not have access to the results, this may not fulfil the obligation which the Vice-Chancellor posited. Medical audit is seen as threatening by some administrators and by some of the public because it is private. Conversely, it is seen as threatening by medical staff to the extent that it is *not* confidential.

The three United Kingdom defence societies, through their co-ordinating secretary, made the following points to the Department of Health in 1990:

> If medical practitioners are to be expected to co-operate wholeheartedly with the audit process (as we are sure they should), it is necessary to explain to them the purposes to which the results of audit might be put and the extent to which confidential information might be made available as a result of the audit process. For example, if it becomes common knowledge that audit reports exist within health authorities which name patients, it is likely that prospective plaintiffs, in seeking discovery of relevant documents under the provisions of the Supreme Court Act 1981, will then also seek discovery of the results of the audit process in the hope of gaining information which might be of assistance in deciding whether or not to initiate litigation for personal injuries or death. Clinicians might also have anxieties about the possibilities of the results of the audit process being used for disciplinary or quasi-disciplinary procedures. The medical defence organisations are keen to support the principles of audit. However, the interests of our members require that adequate consideration be given to a number of sensitive issues arising from the proposed implementation of audit procedures throughout the health services. For example, in some American jurisdictions a degree of legal privilege is afforded to papers generated in the course of audit procedures so that they are not available to prospective plaintiffs. We are advised that, in this country, such privilege is unlikely to extend to records made as part of the audit process and that accordingly such records may be discoverable. We wonder whether your department has given consideration to the possibility of seeking, by statutory process, some form of legal privilege for documents created as a result of the audit procedures and processes.

Sir Donald Acheson replied:

> The question of statutory protection of medical audit data from disclosure in the courts was considered during the preparation of the NHS and Community Care Act 1990, but inclusion of such a clause was not considered appropriate. The Department has agreed with the Joint Consultants Committee to ask the Conference of Medical Royal Colleges to prepare guidance on the issue of confidentiality of audit data.

Professor Aubrey Diamond, Professor of Law at the University of London, advised the Royal College of Physicians' Advisory Committee on Medical Audit in December 1990 that

> it was important to recognise, when considering disclosure of audit documents and legal discoverability, that audit was an education exercise designed to improve standards of patient care, not primarily an exercise in rooting out 'bad apples' ... audit records might be potentially discoverable (and) also be used potentially by employing authorities for disciplinary purposes ....

Professor Diamond indicated that if documents were suspected to exist, the courts could order disclosure. There was little chance that a legal claim of privilege for the documents would succeed in maintaining their confidentiality. The threat of disclosure would have a negative effect on openness in audit meetings. The possibility and desirability of anonymising records were discussed, and the precedent of confidentiality in the first CEPOD report was cited:

> Any audit system has to maintain the highest levels of confidentiality such that the clinicians can be assured they would never be named, sued or otherwise personally denigrated by information contained in the study.[5]

All these working parties have had to deal with reports anonymised with scissors or by blanking out identifying information before photocopying, and with potential problems related to third-party access.

The Scottish Home and Health Department issued a code of practice in September 1990 on the confidentiality of personal health information which included the following:

> The results of medical audit in respect of individual patients and doctors *must remain confidential* at all times.[6] [original emphasis].

It recommended that medical audit reports should not be used for disciplinary purposes and that the Chief Medical Officer should assume the responsibility of ensuring confidentiality of medical audit proceedings. However, there are examples of solicitors acting for plaintiffs who have stipulated in letters-before-action that any clinico-pathological *or audit* reports be identified, locked up and kept safe.

A National Health Service (NHS) circular[7] requires that regular reports be supplied to managers by hospital doctors on the results of medical audit required by the NHS and Community Care Act 1990.

In professional discussions, much stress has been laid on the vulnerability of the doctor to the use of audit reports in litigation against him by a dissatisfied patient or in disciplinary action by a dissatisfied manager. Only more recently has the right of the patient to anonymity and confidentiality been specifically stressed. The same circular specifies that only 'aggregated data or general conclusions' ought to be made available to health authority managers,[7] this being intended to ensure that individual patients are not needlessly identified.

The widely accepted implicit consent of patients to their names and clinical details being made known to medical records departments, pharmacy and other staff on a 'need-to-know' basis cannot be said to apply in the context of audit. If the courts were to classify audit documents as part of a patient's 'medical records', they might be considered to lie within the remit of the Data Protection Act 1984 and the Access to Health Records Act 1990. If it became clear that documents or computerised data had been destroyed after analysis for the purpose of audit, the courts might well be displeased, even though destruction of audit documents has been not only recommended but carried out at the conclusion of many audit studies.

The reporting of untoward incidents and the detection of variations in outcome on a local or national basis are driven by the clinical imperative to improve practice. However, managers need to ensure that audit procedures are being carried out by all health professionals. Public opinion will not tolerate failure to detect dangers. This has become more marked since the introduction of NHS indemnity in January 1990. Following this, apart from collation of financial information about the value of claims paid, there has been little, if any, assessment on the national scale of NHS problems by audit or risk management techniques. A serious problem related to the care of patients may be identified by clinical audit which — if thinly scattered across the country — may be completely missed in the absence of deliberate exercises such as the confidential enquiries into maternal and perioperative deaths and the first CEPOD study.[1]

There is a need for national collation of patterns of 'untoward incidents' and risks on a basis which may have to be given more specific statutory protection from inappropriate disclosure of confidential medical information for any purpose other than audit and prevention of potentially recurring harm.

Even the protection widely assumed to apply to the confidential enquiries into maternal and perioperative deaths has no statutory backing. An inappropriate disclosure, in good faith for a sensible purpose — but nevertheless contrary to the basis on which the information had been contributed — ground the system almost to a halt for some time. Public confidence in the protection of confidentiality will be the vital underpinning of future developments in audit.

References

1. Buck N, Devlin HB, Lunn JN. *First Report of the Confidential Enquiry into Perioperative Deaths.* London: CEPOD, Royal College of Surgeons, 1987
2. Department of Health. *Working for patients.* London: HMSO, 1989

3. Royal College of Surgeons of England. *Guidelines to clinical audit in surgical practice.* London: Royal College of Surgeons, 1989
4. Re. Wilsher v Essex Area Health Authority. TLR 11.3.88 HL
5. Report of Royal College of Physicians. Medical Audit: A second report. London. RCP Publications, 1993
6. Scottish Home and Health Department. Edinburgh: Scottish Home and Health Department, 1990
7. NHS Management Executive Circular HC (91) 2. Medical Audit in the Hospital and Community Health Services. Assuring the Quality of Medical Care: Implementation of Medical and Dental Audit in the Hospital and Community Health Services.

16 | Information technology initiatives of the Information Management Group in relation to clinical audit

Ray Rogers
Head of Information Management Group,
National Health Service Management Executive

The National Health Service Management Executive launched an information management and technology strategy for the NHS in December 1992. Its aim is to enable the NHS to exploit all the potential that information technology can offer.

In forming that strategy, the Information Management Group took advice from a number of people. The Chief Executive's Working Group on Information Management and Technology, formed through an initiative taken by the Conference of Colleges, has proved to be influential so far, and will continue to be important in all the work of the Information Management Group.

The elements of the National Health Service information management and technology strategy

The NHS information management and technology (IM&T) strategy comprises four main initiatives:

1. To put in place a national IM&T infrastructure.
2. To mount national demonstration projects, for example demonstration projects are underway in exploring integrated systems in hospitals (the Hospital Information Support Systems (HISS) project), health care purchasers systems (the Developing Information Systems for Purchasers (DISP) project), community care systems (the Community Information Systems for Providers (CISP) project) and specifications for general practitioner systems.
3. To provide value for money. Investment appraisal, procurement, project management and the like make up this initiative.
4. To develop a human resource strategy for NHS information management and technology staff. This strand will broaden to focus on medical and nursing staff in 1994.

This chapter will concentrate on the infrastructure and outline two of the national demonstration projects, integrated clinical workstations and an electronic patient record.

Nature of the infrastructure

The key principles of the national information management and technology infrastructure are that:

- information systems should be based on information relevant to the clinical care of the patient;
- information for management should be derived from operational systems, from systems used for day-to-day work, and not just for capturing management information;
- systems should be integrated — data should be captured once and, as far as practicable and permissible, shared; and
- information must be secure and confidential, but, subject to appropriate safeguards in relation to confidentiality, should be shared across the NHS.

The main principle is that information systems should be 'person-based', by which is meant that information is held as part of the health record of the individual. Many existing systems are not person-based, but merely capture and count events for managerial purposes. Others, if they capture information on an individual, jettison it after a short period, retaining only counts and information about events. Examples are out-patient booking, pharmacy and many pathology systems, as well as most of the current community systems. Systems such as these, not being person-based, deny the opportunity to link events that happen to an individual within an organisation in order to get a picture of that individual's experience of health care. Similarly, they prevent linking of records across organisations for outcome measurement and clinical audit.

Components of the infrastructure

The National Health Service number

If records are to be held in person-based systems with the potential for linking them, there must be a facility to uniquely identify individuals. The identifier for NHS purposes is to be the NHS number. The existing number has 23 different and inconvenient formats, and is therefore prone to errors in transcription. It has been decided to replace it with an all-numeric, 10-digit number with a check digit. New numbers should be assigned to all the UK population by 1995.

National Health Service administrative registers

A feature of all records is administrative details of individuals: name, address, post-code, NHS number, age, sex, and name of general practitioner. Registers with these details are held by family health service authorities in hospitals, and in the community. They are required by district health authorities and other purchasers. It is wasteful to repeatedly build registers with considerable overlaps and inconsistencies. The Management Executive will be putting in place a system of NHS administrative registers holding these administrative details, designed specifically to allow access by natural communities of sharers, and installed so that they will have national coverage and, in due course, the facility to be linked.

National Health Service-wide electronic networking

An electronic network is required for sharing of patient data, obtaining access to databases such as libraries, outcome databases and administrative registers. Other examples include pathology results, outpatient booking systems, referrals from primary care and discharge letters. The aim is to provide by 1996 an electronic facility enabling any major NHS organisation to communicate with any other by voice and data, including images.

National standards

If electronic access and sharing of information and electronic messaging are to be realised to their full potential, and computers are to be linked, compliance with national standards for interconnections, interworking and messaging will be essential. These standards, which will include data definitions, formats, codes and classifications are being worked out. Compliance with them will be expected throughout the NHS.

Privacy

There needs to be extreme care in respecting the privacy of individuals within this environment of sharing and messaging. Ground rules for safeguarding the confidentiality of personal information are to be issued for consultation. Guidance for preserving confidentiality in the context of contracting has already been promulgated.[1]

Language for health

One of the most challenging aspects of the proposed infrastructure is the intention to create what has become known as a 'language for health'. The data building blocks required for resource management, clinical audit, outcomes, contracting and so on all reside in the patient record. For these purposes, and also (and most importantly) for improved patient care, it is highly desirable to capture electronically at least the essence of the text of the patient record. The way in which this is being developed is outlined in Chapter 13.

Once the dictionary has been created, and the terms or words can be captured from the clinical record, they can be collated and arranged in a variety of ways to serve different purposes. Using the language analogy, they can be grouped in meaningful phrases and sentences. For example, they can be arranged in classifications, like the International Classification of Diseases (ICD.10)[2] or the Office of Population, Censuses and Surveys classification of procedures (OPCS4), into minimum data sets used for contracting or referral, or into iso-resource, iso-need or iso-prognosis groups. The last two types of groups are being considered by the National Case-mix Office.

Of course, the business of health is not just about individuals with a health problem, and thus patients' records, but also about public health, health improvement, disease prevention, health status, health needs and so on. The Read-coded thesaurus of terms and groupings, must therefore — and will — encompass the terms and groupings appropriate to public health.

Capturing the clinical record

In essence, the clinical record contains administrative details, signs and symptoms, the results of investigations, diagnoses and indicators of severity, medicines, therapy, operations, procedures and outcomes. Consultation is under way on national standards for terms in a common administrative data set, and the Read codes will cover the remainder — so there will soon be a full dictionary to encompass all these.

It is necessary to recognise that clinical records have three important features.

1. Records contain a great deal of free text and, with the rapid

technological advances in speech banks, might soon include the spoken word.

2   They will need to have a structured part if it is to be possible to store, analyse, collate, retrieve, group or transmit messages with computers.

3.. There is now an important graphical component, examples of which include images such as X-rays, ultrasound, isotope, computerised tomographic and magnetic resonance scanning, and graphical displays such as ECGs.

The first of the demonstration projects is primarily, but not exclusively, about realising the potential of Read codes and the Clinical Terms Project for capturing text in structured context. The project is concerned with developing the concept of an '*integrated clinical work-station*', developing a computer interface with the doctor, which will facilitate the capture and display of data in a structured way, by displaying appropriate terms from the Read thesaurus.

CASPE Consulting Ltd has reviewed existing initiatives concerned with integrated clinical work-stations and aspects of the electronic patient record.[3] It is planned to demonstrate clinical work-stations in two hospitals in Yorkshire and Scotland, and also take some mobile demonstrators which can be tried in hospitals around the country.

Developing a user-friendly work-station is just one step towards the more difficult problem of *electronically capturing much of the patient record*, which is the object of the other demonstration project — that is, to capture all the structured text, free text, images and graphics, and perhaps voice, which comprise the total record. The objective is to provide the data for patient care, research, resource management audit, outcomes, contracting and management in such a way that all or part of the record is available to authorised carers and others over networks to terminals, wherever they may be. All this must, of course, be subject to strict controls on access for safeguarding the confidentiality of personal data.

There is well established technology to do all this, increasingly cheap computer storage with ever faster access, and computers with more powerful analytical and handling abilities. The problems are not just how to bring all the hardware together but, more important and much more difficult, how best to interface it with doctors and clinicians for use in their everyday business. The additional challenge is to organise that business in a way which exploits that potential to the maximum. We plan to draw on other experience in Europe and the USA.

The United Kingdom is in an excellent position to take on this challenge, albeit a difficult one that will take time. However, if clinicians are to influence the way technology is to be used in their business, *now* is the time to exercise that influence, so that information technology provides what clinicians want.

References

1. National Health Service Management Executive. *Handling confidential patient information in contracting: a code of practice.* EL(92)60
2. Ashley J. International Classification of Diseases: the structure and contents of the 10th revision. *Health Trends* 1991:**22**:135–7
3. CASPE Consulting Ltd. *Review of existing initiatives in the integrated clinical workstation programme.* Report for the NHS Management Executive Information Management Group, 1992

DISCUSSION

Nick Chapman: I am concerned about the new generation of top-down initiatives in information technology. In my experience, no matter how well these are led, they lead to a lack of understanding and commitment when they come to be implemented, used, maintained and, above all, paid for. Clearly, some issues will be resolved only by national initiatives and co-ordination at a national level, but I would be interested to hear views as to whether the balance is right between top-down and bottom-up.

Ray Rogers: We have asked ourselves in what the centre should become involved. Our view is that the NHS Management Executive Information Group should be involved in matters relating to the national infrastructure in information management and technology, and that there cannot be NHS-wide networking without some national, central, involvement. We see the components of the infrastructure outlined on pages 79–80, as areas in which the centre has to be the driving force — albeit, in all the projects, there is a structure which involves users.

What else should the centre do? A training strategy, for example, seems to be a national issue (although we would not do the training).

The most difficult area is that of 'national demonstrator projects' — a phrase I use deliberately. The purpose of these projects is not to design software to be rolled out or to produce some unique way of doing things, but to explore areas that are technologically, organisationally or managerially difficult. Examples of such areas include community systems and the structure of person-based information systems. Therefore, we believe it is proper to explore such issues on two or three different sites in different ways, deliberately opening the doors to everyone, including suppliers, so that we can share in the learning experience.

The development of electronic patient records is another extraordinarily complex area. There will be two large national demonstrators learning from each other and joining with a number of other initiatives around the country which are linked to them.

Linda Patterson: Some issues related to capturing relevant information for the medical record have not been mentioned. For those of us dealing with elderly people and people with chronic disability, their functional capacity and social circumstances, the services they receive, the role of carers, and so on are very real issues which supplement the medical diagnosis, and indeed largely dictate the outcome and use of resources for patients. The clinical management systems so far in existence are not robust in capturing such information. What further work is going on in this regard?

James Read: Because the code originated from general practice and primary care teams, such information has been considered from the start, and is a central part of the Clinical Terms Project. Much of the work of, for example, the Project's working groups in mental health, geriatrics and paediatrics revolves around personal and social information, including information about carers.

Robert Palmer: The benefits of a fully integrated National Health information system are appreciated, but perhaps we have missed the boat to an extent because most units are developing their own clinical or hospital information system on an *ad hoc* basis. Has the timing been wrong for full integration, which now seems a good idea?

Ray Rogers: Many hospitals do not have fully integrated systems yet. Our initiatives have already had a substantial influence on suppliers. Indeed, when HISS started, there were no integrated systems in the market-place, and few suppliers had the relevant experience to be able to offer them. The position has changed markedly now and prices have dropped considerably. Our initiatives have influenced the market-place and will continue to do so.

Section 4

Managers and clinical audit, and resources for audit

17 | The interface between management and clinical audit

David Bowden
Director, Merrett Health Risk Management, Brighton

I begin with four premises, that:

- clinical audit will be of great importance to the fate of the provider organisations;
- clinicians must not be allowed to lose their sense of altruism;
- managers must be involved in clinical audit; and
- it must never be forgotten that an increasing number of managers are clinicians in their own right.

Firstly, clinical audit will be of great importance to the fate of the provider organisations in the revised National Health Service (NHS). They will thrive or fail as much because of the quality of the care they give as of the cost of that care. Furthermore, their success, or otherwise, will depend not only on the quality of the service itself, but on their ability to *prove* that they are providing a good, effective, quality service.

Secondly, most clinicians have a basic sense of altruism about their work, and a genuine desire to prove to themselves and others that they provide an effective service of high quality. In no circumstances should that sense of altruism be allowed to be diminished in any way: rather, management must support it.

The third premise is that until now (and not surprisingly, in view of their huge agenda) managers have largely watched the development of medical and clinical audit from the sidelines. However, in future, managers will not be content to be spectators in this new situation, but will want to be genuine players, in real partnership with clinical colleagues. As Dr Calman writes on p. xiv, if managers are excluded from the audit process, they are unlikely to respond to audit findings in future; if managers *are* involved, they will not fail to respond to such findings.

The fourth premise concerns the definition of 'manager'. Many managers are of course now clinicians. They have a key role to play in audit, alongside their colleagues and the general manager of the organisation. Clinical directors are now vital and senior service managers.

What managers can do for clinical audit

The right environment

Managers have a clear responsibility to create the right environment within the organisation in which clinical audit can thrive. Where it does not exist, they have an obligation to take the lead by giving top-level commitment to support the audit process. Having been involved in trying to promote medical and clinical audit in Brighton Health Authority since 1985, I believe the best approach to this is an evolutionary and non-punitive one, and based on peer review rather than imposition by management. Managers must be positive and pro-active in their actions in promoting this. I also believe that trust boards and health authorities must endorse and be seen to be endorsing and supporting this whole process.

Quality versus quantity

It is also important that trust boards should initiate the debate about quality versus quantity, with doctors involved particularly through the clinical audit process. This debate is the major issue for the NHS, and needs to be addressed by both purchasers and providers. This means asking whether there are any circumstances in the organisation in which we will be prepared knowingly to compromise the quality of care in any particular activity. If so, what are the implications? If not, what are the practical consequences? Does it mean that the quantity of work will need to be reduced? Trusts should be increasingly explicit and specific about this issue. After discussion at the provider level, it also needs to be debated explicitly with the purchasers of care. This is a fundamental issue which, unless addressed, will give rise to a situation in which the patients and staff in a provider unit are placed at significant and continuing risk.

Resources

The third issue is about resources. Effective, let alone comprehensive, clinical audit needs clearly allocated resources to support it, which means the provision of time for clinicians to take part. If it means that some clinics and theatre sessions have to be forfeited, this needs to be openly discussed and acknowledged. The requirement of written job plans is a good opportunity to sort this out.

Resources need to be made available for research and study leave, for information systems, and for the staff to support them, which means both technical and administrative support. Clinical audit should not therefore be seen as a cheap, peripheral activity. It needs time, staff and money to develop in a proper and comprehensive way. Some understanding needs to be reached with the purchasers of care about how much of their money is to be spent on this activity. If they can see the benefits from it, they will be prepared to invest more.

Information Systems

The fourth issue is information systems, which are a key tool in audit — indeed there are encouraging signs that this is being recognised. As patient activity increases, the clinical audit information systems need to be integrated within the corporate information strategy. Currently, different databases support the resource management process and provide the clinical audit data. Working from different information bases makes it much more difficult to create the balance between quality and quantity in clinical departments.

There must be, as Ray Rogers outlines in Chapter 16, much more integration and sharing of the databases. Information produced through the large patient administration systems that support the resource management process is often questioned by clinicians working in individual departments. They do not trust either these or finance and personnel systems to provide them with accurate information. On the other hand, they do own the information from their departmental audit systems. I believe that everything possible must be done to maintain that sense of ownership of the audit information when it eventually forms part of integrated large-scale systems. Ray Rogers stresses the new NHS information strategy built up from individual person-based data, which my experience confirms is very much the right way to move forward.

Incentives

The fifth point is about incentives for clinical audit. If a clinical directorate meets its work-load target, and in doing so does not spend all the money provided by the purchasers, that money can be retained and used for a specific development within the directorate. Managers also need to create some form of incentive system to reward clinicians for achieving improved clinical outcomes, to be measured by audit. The emphasis should be on creating incentives for good work, rather than relying on applying sanctions for poor work.

Techniques of audit

The techniques of clinical audit must also be considered. Managers should help clinicians to develop new techniques, such as occurrence screening, record review, criteria-based audit and measurement of outcomes. There also needs to be a common understanding between managers and clinicians in relation to external accreditation and review.

Patient satisfaction

Managers need to consider measurement of patient satisfaction as part of audit. Patients have a clear understanding about whether or not they are getting a good standard of care in regard to some aspects of a hospital's work. The quality of attention provided in an out-patient department and the arrangements for admitting non-emergency patients are good examples. The clinical audit process helps to create clinical standards on other aspects about which the average patient has little idea as to whether there is good or bad practice. There is a need, therefore, to interface these two elements, so that both what the patient wants and what the patient needs are provided. Clinicians and managers have interlocking roles here.

Guidelines on confidentiality

Finally, managers have a clear obligation, with clinicians, to establish guidelines on confidentiality for the use of medical information, both inside and outside the organisation. There are twin objectives here of preserving clinical confidence, on the one hand, whilst, on the other, using clinical audit information properly, usefully and effectively.

Managers should therefore give a lead in promoting formalised and systematic clinical audit, and provide the necessary support and funding. They should not, however, seek to interfere with individual clinical freedom. Indeed, their aim should be to maximise this, working closely together with clinicians as partners within an agreed system, sharing common values.

What managers need from clinical audit

There are several areas which highlight what managers need from clinical audit and, indeed, will increasingly expect.

Information

Managers both of purchasing authorities and of provider units —
and, indeed, general practitioner fundholders — need information
to determine the quality of clinical services. Increasingly, they will
want to assess which activities and treatments provide the most
effective outcomes. I believe that managers should be drawn into
the identification and agreement of clinical protocols and standards, and must also be involved in comparing predicted and actu-
al outcomes of activity, in partnership with the clinicians concerned.*

Information is also needed to assess how well a clinical audit process is working, and therefore meeting the objective of providing
better patient care. Managers will continue to invest in audit only if
it results in some positive benefits for patients, and is generally seen
to be improving patient care.

Contracting

Secondly, there will be increasing pressure from purchasers to
establish progressively more advanced quality standards in service
contracts. As contracting skills develop, there needs to be discussion about whether purchasers will want to have information about
clinical outcome measures or merely some evidence that clinical
audit meetings are taking place.

Treatment standards

Purchasers will probably want to see some evidence that specific
treatment standards are being met, and providers should not make
this difficult for them. On the other hand, if providers are not
careful, they will find the whole process being purchaser-driven.
Clinical audit has been traditionally provider-led, and it should stay
that way. Clinicians must therefore be involved in establishing
some of the quality standards in contract specifications, which
should be relate quality to work-loads and costs.

Co-ordinated approaches

Provider chief executives will want to see a more co-ordinated
approach to managing resources and work-load, on the one hand,

---

*Editor's note: A recent NHS Executive letter (EL (93) 115) lays out how purchasers should
use clinical guidelines in contracting.

and assuring the quality of services, on the other. Clinical directors are the key to ensuring the totally integrated management of quality, quantity, cost and accessibility, the four key elements in the contracting process. In some situations, the clinical director is responsible for the management of resources, with one of his colleagues taking responsibility for co-ordinating the clinical audit programme. I believe that the clinical director increasingly needs to lead both. Although trust clinical audit committees have a key role to play in stimulating, encouraging and supporting clinical audit throughout the organisation, the processes must be owned by the individual clinical departments. It needs to be devolved (and seen to be devolved) increasingly down to the line managers — the clinical directors. Clinical audit and resource management must be co-ordinated in a patient-centred directorate in order to achieve a more cost-effective service.

Involvement of all health professionals

The fourth important issue here is the involvement of *all* health professionals in audit leading to a patient-related focus. It is legitimate and necessary for medical audit to continue in its own right, but increasingly there must be more interprofessional audit because this also creates a greater joint understanding of potentially high-risk situations.

Risk management

Crown indemnity for medical negligence was introduced on 1 January 1990. Providers are now responsible for initially funding the consequences of such negligence. Huge sums of money are being spent on meeting these costs, and are therefore not available for direct patient care. Risk management and prevention can significantly reduce the costs of adverse clinical events, some of which lead to claims of negligence. Risk management should be regarded as an essential part of any system of quality management. It improves the quality of patient care by assessing in advance, and trying to evaluate, identified risks or, once adverse events have happened, taking some positive action to eliminate or reduce the likelihood of their future recurrence.

Risk management extends beyond clinical audit as it is concerned with factors outside the purely clinical fields. Most untoward incidents do not occur as a result of a single clinician making a single mistake. Many result from a number of small mistakes coming together to form a significant adverse event. Outside the NHS, the King's Cross underground fire disaster was a good example. More significantly, most adverse events occur as a result of a systems failure, often involving people and services outside the direct clinical team: for example, breakdowns in communication between professionals and with patients, people working beyond their competence, staff having ill-defined responsibilities relative to their colleagues, and clinicians in the same team working to different clinical protocols.

There needs to be a more pro-active approach to managing untoward occurrences and incidents. There is a definite need for better systems for early warning of risks and of reporting adverse events. We must be more open and honest with patients if something goes wrong. This will help reduce the number of claims of negligence.

Conclusion

Clinical audit will be of increasing importance to the success and viability of provider units. Managers and clinicians must work more closely together. Doctors should maximise the tremendous opportunities available to them to be more involved in shaping and organising the provider services, and managers should become better educated and better informed about the work of their clinical colleagues. The joint initiative of the Royal College of Physicians and the Institute of Health Service Management in running courses on medicine for managers is a good way forward.

18 | Management's legitimate interests in clinical audit

Peter Coe
District General Manager, East London and The City Health Authority

The establishment of general management in the National Health Service (NHS) clearly invests full responsibility in one person for the management of the organisation. Thus, management must be interested in any internal process which influences the organisation. If this process concerns core standards and underlying principles of the management of resources, it would be expected that managers would show a keen interest. The agenda for implementing *The health of the nation*[1] includes identifying ways of achieving a unified NHS for our patients with no barrier between primary and secondary care. Clinical audit must therefore be undertaken in such a way as to lead to joint protocols and guidelines between primary and secondary health care professionals, and joint measurement of outcomes.

Assessment of health needs

If purchasers of health care look not only at *The health of the nation* but at needs assessment in general terms for a local population, how can they do this without any input from clinical audit? From a review of the published literature, public health colleagues and managers can access a vast range of information and ideas about the direction the organisation should take and what the strategy for health care should be. This needs to be interpreted for each locality. In Tower Hamlets, for example, seven neighbourhoods have been identified, so we think increasingly not just of one particular organisation but of seven. With the fusion of commissioning authorities in East London, there will clearly be far more than seven localities or communities, each with their different characteristics needing a different approach. In working with general practitioners locally, and identifying the commissioning needs for their particular communities, feedback is needed from all the health professionals locally about the way in which different needs are to be met.

Organisational assessment

General management spends much of its time comparing performance, both across and within organisations. Performance indicators have demonstrated the value of comparing year-on-year internally, which cannot be done unless professional staff can be relied on constantly to compare professional performance. If the organisation itself needs to learn and to change, the rapport between professional staff and management must be such that the outcomes of assessment can be considered together.

Resource utilisation

In purchasing health care, managers and clinicians alike constantly assess value for money. If outcomes will be purchased at the same price but different in terms of quality of process, this must influence the way in which commissioning future health care is considered. General practitioner fundholders, however informally, are certainly influenced by outcome and by their own audit assessments of their secondary care professional colleagues.

Risk management

Chapter 17 outlines some of the principles of risk management and the need for safe systems of care. Management has legitimate interests in ensuring that there is the least possible legal action because its value in cash terms can be better invested in good health care. Management's legitimate interest is that the organisation offers the best standards for each individual cared for by that organisation.

Investment for change

The NHS market now allows more freely than previously the opportunity to plan for changes in referral patterns. General practitioner fundholders probably use this freedom more than district or family health service authorities, but dialogues between management and primary care referrers increasingly ask questions about the ability of providers to deliver the required standards.

As services change, both purchasing and providing managers will need to ask questions about the impact of investment. Managers need assurance that professional staff have confidence in their ability to respond to new challenges, and can advise management on the appropriate nature of the investment required. Too many hospital store-rooms are full of 'wonderful' equipment that has never been used.

In considering investment in a cash-limited NHS, management must be reassured about its present use of resources. It is legitimate, therefore, that both purchasing and providing managers should be interested in what can be learnt from clinical audit about the appropriate use of resources. If managers can show that their organisation is at least as efficient as comparable organisations, they can negotiate for more resources from a position of strength.

Managers must also be interested in effectiveness: that is, the perceived added value delivered to the health of a patient or to a service by the use of a resource. Systems or procedures are often changed — only to be changed back again because they prove to be of less value or there is no perceivable difference.

On arrival in Tower Hamlets, I was told that the most outstanding issue was that of mental health. There was general agreement on this — there still is, but it is as yet undecided how to resolve the issue. Despite numerous professional assessments, there is not agreement on the right way forward. Mental health professionals advised the establishment of a day hospital for mental health. All the capital and revenue costs were identified, we were all set to go, but no one could say how many patients would be treated or what added value the day hospital would make to their lives; in other words, we might be planning to follow 'good practice', but it had not been demonstrated that any value was likely to be added by that investment to any person's mental health.

Working with other agencies

How clinical audit will work externally to professions outside the NHS needs to be considered. New systems of care opened up by 'Care in the community'[2,3] may result in real problems in discharge arrangements. Feedback is needed from the different professions, particularly from clinical audit, into the appropriateness of how residents of Tower Hamlets receive care. I shall be challenged if standards of care in Tower Hamlets are not acceptably in line with those elsewhere.

It is in my interest that purchasers from across the country will want to buy services from hospitals and community services in Tower Hamlets because it reduces the unit price. This means that standards of care in my local unit should be as high, if not higher, than anywhere else. I want to work with the provider units to ensure that this is the case.

There are three principal tasks for NHS managers — to identify issues in the NHS, to ensure that people are available who can resolve those issues, and to ensure that the environment is correct for these people to work in. Clinical audit must be at the top of any manager's agenda when tackling any of these issues.

References

1. Department of Health. *The health of the nation — a strategy for health in England.* London: HMSO; 1992
2. Secretaries of State for Health, Social Security and Wales. *Caring for people: Community care in the next decade and beyond.* London: HMSO, 1989
3. Groves T ed. *Countdown to community care.* London: BMJ publications, 1993

DISCUSSION

Russell Hopkins: In discussing what managers want from audit, complaints were not mentioned. As part of their quality initiative, managers are increasingly seeking to use clinical audit as a way of monitoring complaints.

I do not believe that the director of clinical services should also chair the audit committee. It is crucial that the former remain clinicians, and give enough time to do their clinical services and also undertake management functions. A director of clinical services in an average district general hospital has a big (and sufficient) job. If they also chair audit committees, their clinical services will suffer. More importantly, the director of clinical services is part of line management, in a line relation to the general manager. In my view, clinical audit must be separate. It is a professional activity and service, independent of purchaser and provider. In a trust situation, if a clinical director held both roles and audit discovered that contracts were not doing well and quality was low, it would be easy to hide this. The chairman of the audit committee should have enough time to do the job properly, and not be in line management.

David Bowden: I believe that there is a clear managerial responsibility for the management of resources on behalf of the clinical director to the chief executive, probably directly or perhaps through the director of clinical services. On the other hand, audit should be seen to be, and actually be, a genuine peer review activity for which the clinical director should be accountable, in that sense, to his colleagues. I do not think these two things are in conflict, but need to come together increasingly — because increasingly when we talk about money, we should talk about quality, and vice versa. Unless one person in a clinical department is focusing on that, it is more difficult to get a genuine and sensible discussion.

Peter Coe: When commissioning authorities become larger, as is happening in East London, my commissioning colleagues and I will want to discuss with local clinicians coronary heart disease, disability, ophthalmology, etc. This will bring together people from different provider units to advise commissioners about the right way forward for standards of care. It may mean that commissioners will be negotiating with somebody not necessarily working in a line management relationship to the chief executive of a trust, and that they have to say things not necessarily in the interests of that trust. It will be a testing time for all of us to steer a professional path through these relationships.

David Moss: How can we learn from mistakes and disasters, from complaints, and from cases that go to litigation?

David Bowden: Most clinical negligence actions result from failures of systems rather than of individuals. We need to be much more pro-active in identifying the potential for risk. I believe this identification depends on thinking about things differently, changing both attitudes and behaviour in certain circumstances. For example, when will there be the first Suzy Lamplugh case in general practice or community district nursing — and what will we do when it happens?* Why not do something now, instead of waiting for it to happen — or at least analyse the risks and determine whether anything can be done?

There also needs to be a more open attitude within our organisations, whether in primary care or in an acute teaching hospital, so that managers would feel able to say to all their staff 'I want to make a deal with you: whenever you make a mistake, when something has gone wrong, please tell me immediately and ask what can be done about it. In return, I will not seek to pillory, discipline or dismiss you, provided that you have not gone beyond the rules. I want to use our problems positively.'

The response I often receive to this is: do I want people to 'tell' on a colleague if they see him or her making a mistake? I believe that anyone in an organisation with a proper level of openness and honesty (which managers should increasingly try to encourage) should report any mistake that is identified — which does not necessarily mean 'telling' on people. After all, why are we here, and

---

*Editor's note: Suzy Lamplugh was a female estate agent who disappeared in London, probably murdered by a client to whom she was showing a property.

what are we trying to do? Do we want to cover up mistakes or bring them out in the open and use them in a beneficial way?

Richard Wray: We have had to consider a related problem recently. For some years we have had a fairly open system of reporting mistakes, deliberately writing down little or nothing. The stage has now been reached where we are considering whether to have a written system, at least for the more important incidents. A form has been produced internally for that purpose, for trial use by medical staff alone rather than widely in clinical audit. What is your view about this?

David Bowden: It is quite simple to devise techniques that cope with anonymous reporting, but I hope a more open situation can be achieved.

We also need to consider how honest and open we are with patients when something has gone wrong. We need to be able to tell them about it, to say that they should be the first to know, and that *this* particular step has been taken, the cause has been identified, certain things have been stopped so that it will not happen again, and *these* are the results of the initial investigation. We should say that a fuller explanation will be given later.

What is so irritating for a manager is that these mistakes are not reported. Two years later a letter is received from a solicitor, and we know that any litigation cannot be defended because of the inadequacy of the medical, nursing and surgical records. Management and patients must be informed immediately — the latter then feel better about it and less angry.

Russell Hopkins: In California and elsewhere in the USA, hospital managers have discovered that the open reporting of untoward incidents has reduced the number both of clinical errors and of doctors being sued. A system of untoward incident reporting must be open to all members of the hospital staff, not just doctors and nurses but to everybody, because many people are involved in care in peripheral ways as well as directly.

Patrick Jeffery: For about two years we have had a system of reporting of untoward incidents based entirely on anonymous reporting from any member of the staff about any aspect that he or she thinks might be critical or untoward. Clinical directors and the audit department are jointly involved.

Peter Coe: A distinction has to be made between what is an appropriate clinical audit enquiry staying within the professions, and when external bodies. should be involved. A patient in my last health authority died in a mental health unit. We had a thorough investigation, but we could not be open about it because the police were investigating potential murder or manslaughter. Six months later, another patient had her arm broken in the same mental health unit during forcible restraint. No untoward incident was reported. I found out only by an anonymous letter eight to nine weeks later. The culture in that unit was alien to sharing and to honesty. There have been further incidents since then, and I feel that only by having a partnership can the situation be improved. Another aspect that must also be considered is when should the medical profession invoke 'the three wise men' approach, rather than keeping the problem within audit?

Patricia Kent: Another point for discussion in terms of the outcomes of audit is that, as far as trusts are concerned, managers who do not take care of problems highlighted by audit (such as a lack of resource to provide an adequate service) are potentially subject to corporate liability. When clinicians indicate that a major problem could occur, managers would be well advised to take notice of it.

19 | The role and training of audit co-ordinators and audit assistants

Patricia Kent
Regional Audit Co-ordinator, Yorkshire Regional Health Authority and Chair, Medical Audit Association

The primary role of audit staff is to support clinicians in their audit activities. The title in general use is audit assistant, but audit staff would prefer the terms audit facilitator, adviser, officer or analyst.

Some audit staff are able to undertake necessary field work such as literature searches for evidence of effectiveness and to find sources for clinical guidelines. They collect, analyse and interpret data. Many of them present the results of audit to clinicians, and set in train the necessary administrative work to implement changes in clinical practice.

In addition to managing other audit staff, audit co-ordinators provide administrative support to the chairman of the audit committee, work with health professionals who still have not taken much interest in audit, and liaise with others concerned with quality assurance. Many audit co-ordinators are expected to manage the budget, write business plans for the department, and write the annual report for the regional health authority.

Background and training of audit staff

A report from Brunel University showed that the backgrounds of audit staff were medical secretarial or medical records (40%), nursing 32%, information technology or computing 8%, and medicine 3%. It also showed that 29% of audit staff had not been offered any basic training to do the job, and over 50% felt that their training had been inadequate or barely adequate.[1]

The Medical Audit Association has also surveyed audit staff and, as a result, felt that the type of training most needed was entry-level basic audit training undertaken as soon as possible after starting the job. Table 1 lists the components of a three- or five-day basic training course.

Audit staff have identified a further group of courses which

Table 1. Topics for consideration in the training of audit staff

---

Theory and principles of clinical audit
Relationship of clinical audit to other quality assurance activities
Medical terminology
Defining objectives for an audit
Methods of audit
Design of questionnaires and proformas
How to search the medical literature and how to appraise it
The differences between audit and research
Information services and resources
Information systems and coding
Information handling and uses of computers (but not instruction on how
    to use a computer)
Statistics
Basic presentation skills
Content of audit reports
Legal issues — confidentiality
              — Data Protection Act
Current clinical audit initiatives
Latest initiatives of the Department of Health
Working with audit committees
Support networks

---

should be offered within one year of appointment. This coincides both with an increased awareness of the requirements of the job which generally starts at about six months in post, and with a need to be aware of current initiatives that might influence clinicians' decisions in choice of audit topics.

Audit staff would also like to improve their skills in interpreting medical articles, so that they might both provide useful ideas about clinical guidelines and also better recognise and evaluate reports of good practice. They would like to have periodic updates on current thinking on aspects of confidentiality and the uses of audit in risk management.

In addition, some audit staff may need, depending on their background, training in assertiveness and stress management. Audit officers on Grade 3 salaries are frequently in the position of trying to persuade reluctant doctors to audit. As to stress management, stress is *not* created by the unceasing demand from clinicians for audit and the rush of managers to verify quality improvement, but rather from having to deal with a variety of sometimes reluctant clinicians and difficult management issues.

Training for clinical audit co-ordinators

Training for audit co-ordinators (the more senior post) should include basic management skills and continuing education in issues impinging on audit (Table 2). Audit co-ordinators find that once they begin training in business planning many other problems are naturally resolved. They learn more about setting budgets and assessing the needs of their staff for training and so on. A business plan for the department is a useful tool, and also enables appropriate costing for audit and services in contracts.

Through increased awareness of research and development strategy, knowledge of epidemiology and standard setting, co-ordinators, will be able to develop their advisory role. Through continued updating of purchasers' needs, and regional *Health of the nation* strategies,[1] co-ordinators will be able to suggest suitable topics for audit.

Co-ordinators would like to be better at managing change, especially by influencing health professionals to audit, getting more systematic audit through a specialty, and working on issues with contracts and commissioning. Well-trained audit staff should be seen as the way in which clinicians' decisions on changes in practice can

Table 2. Topics for consideration in the training of clinical audit co-ordinators

---

Multidisciplinary and multiprofessional clinical audit

Liaison and integration with other quality initiatives

Writing objectives for audit, and helping set standards

Research skills and their application

Issues relating to service specification, monitoring contracts, and communication with management and purchasers

The uses of audit within the current quality initiatives
   — *The patient's charter*
   — *The health of the nation*

Outcome indicators and health status assessment

Influencing and persuading skills, and managing change

Assertiveness, and 'selling' the audit department

Presentation skills

Managing time and stress

Support networks

Budget setting and business planning

(In addition, some of the topics listed in Table 1 covered at a more advanced level)

---

be fed back to all those people who are relevant to the service, so that change can be rapidly implemented.

There is much concern about the uses of audit in relation to contracts and current quality initiatives such as *The patient's charter*.[2] Audit staff feel that they are the most appropriate staff to undertake the continued structure audits for *The patient's charter* so that correct sampling techniques are used. Many districts in Yorkshire audit discharge plans and work with community care colleagues, ready for the implications of *The patient's charter* and the NHS and Community Care Act 1990.

Terms of employment

Short-term contracts are a major problem. Initially, many staff were on six-month or one-year contracts. Managers feel it is uneconomical to pay for training with such short-term contracts. There is also concern at the lack of recognised structure within provider units, and about the wide variation in titles, job descriptions, and grades across regional health authorities.

Accountability

One way to determine management's commitment to quality of clinical care is to look at the line management of audit co-ordinators. We believe that there is little true commitment to quality if the line manager is a medical records manager or an information manager. Audit staff should be under the direction of the director of clinical services.

Career paths

What are the career paths for audit staff? They can return to their original profession in a managerial role, or make a lateral move to a quality assurance department. The Medical Audit Association has ten ex-audit officer members who now work for purchasing departments as 'intelligence officers'. Audit staff could become directors of quality within a provider or purchasing group, or move into general management.

Conclusion

People coming into the field of clinical audit need basic training, agreement on continuing education (a major component of all quality management programmes) and a proper career structure, perhaps reflected in a national vocational qualification. Audit staff would like to increase their advisory role. They believe that they are (or will become) the experts in audit. They would also like to help implement change.

References

1. Department of Health. *The health of the nation — a strategy for health in England.* London: HMSO, 1992
2. Department of Health. *The patient's charter.* London: HMSO, 1991

20 | How well are audit committees working?

Anthony Hopkins
Research Unit, Royal College of Physicians of London

Guidance about the introduction and membership of district medical audit committees was provided in a health service circular.[1] After the enactment of the NHS and Community Care Act 1990, and the separation of the purchase from the provision of care, audit committees were left to some extent in limbo, uncertain as to whether they should relate to the purchaser or to the provider function. There was also concern, as David Colin-Thome writes on page 20, that a great deal of clinical audit activity has been driven by thoughts such as 'what sort of committee should we set up?', rather than being the natural process of health professionals simply undertaking audit.

I chair the audit working group of the Conference of Medical Royal Colleges and their Faculties in the United Kingdom, and am therefore in a position to hear the uncertainties expressed about the function of audit committees — so I decided to find out what was going on.

Questionnaire survey of audit committees

Based upon my own experience of chairing a district medical audit committee and from a number of conversations with colleagues and publications, I devised a proforma.* This asked for some factual information, such as the membership of local audit committees, and also for some qualitative information about the difficulties and successes encountered in the early years of medical audit, now subsumed into clinical audit.

I wrote to all regional audit leads, and asked for a list of chairpersons of the audit committees known to them. Even this initial step took some time, as the lists proved surprisingly difficult to obtain. Of the 246 committee chairmen and women who were

---

*Copies are available from the Publications Department, Royal College of Physicians.

identified and were asked to complete the questionnaires, 187 replied. Of these, 86 (46%) considered themselves to be chairmen or women of district medical audit committees, 63 (34%) of NHS trusts, and 38 (20%) of directly managed units. However, comments written on a number of the forms indicated that many chairs were uncertain both as to the constitution of their own audit committees, and also whether they reflected purchaser or provider audit functions.

The membership of the 187 medical audit committees is outlined in Table 1. It proved to be encouraging, in the context of this book, insofar as post-graduate tutors and managers were commonly represented. I was, however, surprised by the low number of members of professions allied to medicine — which will undoubtedly change as we move rapidly to clinical audit.

The most frequent specialty of the chairman or woman of the audit committee was anaesthetics (21), closely followed by general surgery (20), geriatric medicine (13) and general medicine and paediatrics (each with 12.) Nearly all the other specialties were represented, but it was surprising to identify only one public health physician chairman of a medical audit committee. I had thought that public health medicine would take a lead in audit, acting as a bridge for ensuring the provision of quality care to the patients in their purchasing locality.

Table 1. Members of 187 medical audit committees

Profession	No. of members
General practitioners	194
Consultant physicians	286
Consultant surgeons	269
Consultant obstetricians	133
Public health physicians	155
Consultants in other specialities	776
The (medically qualified) directors of clinical services	62
Post-graduate tutors	182
Junior doctors	99
Senior nurses	57
Physio/occupational speech therapists	8
Audit co-ordinators/managers	181
Other managers	129
Community health council representatives	8
Other lay persons	20

In response to a question about the administrative support available for the audit committee, 73% of the 179 respondents said that the support was very good, 22% fair, and only 5% poor.

Consultant sessions were paid for in the case of 61% of the 175 respondents, but the other 31% took on this responsibility out of their clinical time; 8% did not respond to this question.

Table 2 shows who received the minutes of the medical audit committee. In the context of this book, it is encouraging that the general manager or chief executive of the trust had access to the minutes in 100 of the 187 cases. It was surprising, however, that only 56 (30%) of district health authorities saw the minutes of the most important committee which concerned the quality of care provided in their district. This low proportion could of course reflect the move to locating audit more firmly in the provider units.

Another question was whether any audits had been commissioned by the trust or other provider unit management, or by health authorities. Only 30% of chairs had been requested to undertake audits suggested by managers. There was virtually no resistance to the concept of commissioned audits.

Part of the drive behind the NHS reforms was to involve users more in the choices of health care that might be provided. It is interesting that only 4 (2%) of 178 respondents to this question reported that the local community health council had requested an audit. (Reference to Table 1 also shows the small number of community health council representatives on audit committees.)

If patients complain about their care, there is an *a priori* case that it may have been of less good quality than it could have been. It would be thought that such complaints would be of interest to medical audit committees, but 87% of 170 respondents to an enquiry about this reported that complaints were not seen by the

Table 2. Who receives the minutes of the medical audit committees?

Recipient of minutes	No. receiving minutes
Trust/provider unit medical staff committee	97
Trust/provider unit general manager or chief executive	100
Trust/provider unit quality assurance committee	42
District health authority in which lies the trust or provider unit	56

(The total is greater than the number of questionnaires returned as more than one box was checked by many of the 187 respondents.)

audit committee, a further 9% received only a summary of the complaints, and only 4% reported viewing all complaints by patients.

The system of complaints within the NHS is now under review by a working group chaired by Professor Alan Wilson. No doubt consideration will be given to simplifying the present disparate and complex procedures, and perhaps also to a better integration of the complaints and clinical audit procedures within a hospital.

It was disappointing that at the time of completion of the questionnaires more than $3\frac{1}{2}$ years after the publication of the White Paper, *Working for patients*,[2] 53 (30%) of the 177 audit committees that responded to this question had had no contact with their local medical audit advisory group.

At the time of the questionnaire survey, and until the end of the financial year 1993–94, audit has been funded by a ring-fenced allocation from the Department of Health to regions, and thence to district health authorities. At the introduction of the system, districts had no option as to the proportion of funds that they could spend on capital or on revenue, this being determined by central financial controls. I therefore asked the chairs of the audit committees how they had spent the allocated capital. Most reported that the money had been spent on stand-alone computer systems, but several reported that the capital budget for audit had been subsumed into the information technology budget of the district or hospital as a whole. Other capital had been spent on office furniture and structural alterations to accommodate audit co-ordinators and audit assistants. Other districts had employed management consultants, or had spent money on library searches, distance learning packages, conferences, projection equipment and so on. A number of respondents reported that they had been unsuccessful in obtaining funds for audit from their local finance department, despite ring-fenced capital being available.

A disappointing feature of the survey was an overwhelming criticism of finance departments, not only in sometimes not being able to obtain allocated capital from them as already indicated, but also in the delayed release of capital, so that it was impossible to plan ahead without knowing how much the capital would be. Many health service managers appear to have the perception that ring-fenced audit money could be used for other purposes. Conversely, some audit committee chairpersons felt that the arbitrary division between revenue and capital is inappropriate, and that capital was unwisely and hastily spent on unproven computer systems before adequate systems of audit had been worked out (a view that I share).

With regard to revenue expenditure, most respondents understandably reported that their principal expenditure was on salaries and training costs for audit staff. The licensing and maintenance of computer software was a further frequently mentioned item. Creative accountancy allowed some districts and hospitals to feel that they could use the audit money to contribute to the running costs of their post-graduate medical centre. Others required the audit budget to be used for upgrading record retrieval from the medical records department, and for photocopying charges. Chairmen and women were sometimes critical of how the revenue was spent, one hospital manager reportedly insisting that no less than £13,750 per annum, out of a total budget of £110,000, was spent on a computer maintenance contract.

Audit activities within hospitals were also covered in the questionnaire. Table 3 shows the frequency of audit meetings, the modal frequency being every two months, but 40% of all respondents reported audit meetings at intervals of three months or greater.

More than half (53%) of the 179 respondents to a question about the times of audit meetings reported that they were held at unsocial hours, and nearly three-quarters (74%) reported that clinical work was regularly displaced by audit meetings. If clinical audit is to be, as I believe it should, a normal part of the working week, meetings should not be held at unsocial hours, but equally it has to be accepted that clinical work such as a routine outpatient clinic or a theatre session will necessarily be displaced by an audit meeting. Clinicians are in a difficult situation: they neither want to cancel clinical activities, nor do they want to hold audit meetings at unsocial hours. This 'bind' probably accounts for the figure just cited of

Table 3. Frequency of medical audit meetings

Frequency of meetings	No. of meetings (%)
More often than monthly	1 (0.6)
Monthly	37 (21)
Every two months	66 (37)
Every three months	58 (33)
Every four months	9 (5)
Less often than every four months	3 (2)
Other	3 (2)
Total respondents	177 (100)

40 per cent of clinicians reporting audit meetings at intervals of three months or greater.

Colleagues were asked to report any audits that had a substantial impact upon clinical practice in their hospitals. There was an encouragingly large number of reports, ranging from improvements in the management of myocardial infarction to a better policy for the use of laxatives. It was also encouraging that 97% of all respondents reported participation in one or more national audits carried out under the auspices of the Colleges.

Clinicians were also asked how they perceived the additional pressures of audit. The 168 chairmen and women of the audit committees who replied reported that their perception was that their local clinicians felt greatly pressed in 15% of instances, and pressed in a further 60%. The figures were similar for the junior doctors, 15% being perceived to be greatly pressed by the requirements of audit, and 56% pressed.

Table 4 shows who does the audits. A small number of districts and hospitals employ commercial firms to undertake audits on their behalf. Consultants and junior medical staff seem to be playing a reasonable part in audit.

Many colleagues had expressed concerns to me about the difficulties in retrieving medical records for audits, so some structured questions were included in the questionnaire (such as those shown in Table 5). The questions were obviously misunderstood by some respondents, as the total number of responses to this question exceeds the total number of questionnaires returned. None the less, the overall pattern of responses suggests continuing difficulties in medical records departments in providing case notes for audit purposes. As already noted, some records departments charged

Table 4. Who does audits?

Participants in audit	Yes	No
	No.	No.
Junior medical staff	157	13
Consultants and their secretaries in the course of routine work	146	24
Clinicians specifically paid to undertake audits	22	27
Audit assistants employed by district/trust/provider unit	162	9
External commercial firms	14	135

(The total is greater than the number of questionnaires returned as more than one box was checked by many respondents.)

Table 5. Retrieval of medical records

Quality of medical record retrieval	No.	%
1. Patients' diagnoses and procedures are accurately coded. Selection of patients from a computer database with a particular diagnosis is easy, and their clinical records can be readily retrieved for manual audit reviews.	49	24.3
2. As (1), but indices of severity of illness and quality are also available in the database.	3	1.5
3. Information systems are limited, and a fair amount of manual sorting needs to be carried out before a suitable sample of records is available for review.	72	35.6
4. As (3), but coding is also deficient.	37	18.3
5. As (4), but there are serious deficiencies in retrieving written records due to staffing and other difficulties in the medical records department.	41	20.3

audit budgets for retrieving records. Partial retrieval of a series of records for audit purposes will seriously bias the results. As a simple example, it is well recognised that the case notes of patients who have been transferred to another hospital for further care, or who have died, are often missing from the records department.

Respondents were also asked whether they had encountered any problems relating to confidentiality. In general, there were remarkably few concerns about confidentiality, and 89% of 179 respondents had not encountered any problems. The Conference of Medical Royal Colleges and their Faculties in the United Kingdom has published guidelines about access to medical records for the purposes of medical audit[3] (John Wall considers the issues further in Chapter 15.)

The primary function of clinical audit is to improve the quality of care provided to patients, and, as such, must be firmly linked to the post-graduate training of all health professionals. It is disappointing, therefore, that more than one-third (36%) of 178 respondents replied negatively to a question as to whether audit was firmly linked to post-graduate education. Various qualitative comments in relation to this question suggest that the links between audit activities and post-graduate education are not robust, a great deal depending upon the enthusiasm of the local clinical tutors. One respondent remarked that in his hospital, the audit office was situated in the post-graduate centre, which seems an idea worthy of consideration by others.

Conclusion

It has been possible to present only a small fraction of the enormous amount of information gathered from the questionnaire survey. However, some overall conclusions can be drawn.

First, there are some encouraging points. Audit is well established, most clinicians now recognise the need for audit, and many are participating in regional and national audits. There are few concerns about issues of confidentiality, and most health professionals would welcome audits suggested by purchasers, provider unit managers, or users of health services.

However, there remain a number of concerns. Many consultants remain unenthused about the advantages of audit, and concerned both about how time and resources taken for audit may displace medical activity and also about the rigour of the methods by which audit is pursued. Links between hospital audit and audit in the primary care sector remain weak, and links with post-graduate education are not yet robust. There remains a lack of clarity about where audit committees sit between purchasers and providers, and indecision about the right size for a committee.

When the conference on which this book is based was held, there was concern about the future funding of medical audit. The focus of the Department of Health has rapidly moved towards clinical audit, and ring-fenced funding will terminate at the end of the financial year 1994–95.[4] Thereafter, in England and Wales there will be no further central allocation to regions for audit, and purchasers and providers together will have to negotiate prices which will include quality assurance activities, including clinical audit. There are obvious concerns here. For example, a provider may tender for a contract at a low price, first, because his care is not of such a good quality as another provider's, and secondly, because he does not plan to spend money on measuring quality anyway. It is therefore absolutely essential that purchasers recognise that they must build into their contracts quality measures that can be audited, and be prepared to pay for that auditing and monitoring function.

Difficulties can be foreseen even if this course is followed. For example, a purchaser may be prepared to supplement the 'raw' contract price by adding on a 5% supplement for audit purposes. However, if a clinical directorate such as cardiological services keeps all its 5% for auditing cardiological services, there will be no audit monies available for auditing the institutional structure of a provider unit as a whole, for example, how it looks after acute medical admissions. It may be that provider unit management will need to top-slice the proportion of all contracts for central audit functions. This problem is currently being considered by the Department of Health's Clinical Outcomes Group. In whatever way it is decided to fund audit, purchasing and provider unit managers must make explicit the budget available for audit purposes, and release the money in a timely manner so that audit committees and audit co-ordinators can plan ahead.

The relationship between clinical audit and the central hospital information system also requires further development. My judgement is that 'clinical audit systems', so heavily marketed in the early years of audit, should now be a thing of the past. Improved connectivity between personal computers and central patient administration systems should mean that the data collected for operational management of clinical problems of individual patients can be collected once only on central systems, and the resulting database questioned in a variety of ways by personal computers within clinical directorates. Clinicians need to determine small data sets of clinically relevant information that should be stored, and measures of case severity and comorbidity, and also work harder at defining outcomes other than mortality.

The theme of this book is the interrelationship between professional activity within the health service and the managers of the health service. This chapter has concentrated on the difficulties encountered by clinicians, but managers also will have difficulties if the information they receive about audit is restricted to anonymised brief and uninformative minutes of audit meetings. Unless they have been fully involved at an early stage, managers are also unlikely to respond to requests for more resources to improve the service thought to be deficient as a result of an audit.

References

1. Department of Health. HC (91) 2. Medical Audit in the Hospital and Community Health Services. Assuring the Quality of Medical Care: Implementation of Medical and Dental Audit in the Hospital and Community Health Services.
2. Department of Health. *Working for patients.* London: HMSO, 1989
3. Conference of Medical Royal Colleges and their Faculties in the United Kingdom. Access to medical records for the purposes of medical audit. *British Medical Journal* 1992; **306**: facing page 913
4. NHS Management Executive. Clinical audit in HCHS: allocation of funds 1993/94. EL (93) 34

DISCUSSION

Charles Shaw: There are practical problems in retrieving medical records for medical audit. It takes a lot of time to retrieve large numbers of records—and somebody has to pay for it. I believe it is legitimate that some of the audit money is used for this purpose.

The other issue is the responsibility of clinicians in contributing to clinical records, in particular in recording diagnoses, procedures, outcomes and complications. It is impossible for any computer system to retrieve the information — no matter how well it is driven or how well trained the coding staff. It would be valuable if the audit working group of Conference or the Clinical Outcomes Group could give some guidance on exactly whose job it is to write what, and where.

Anthony Hopkins: Storing and retrieving medical records are functions of a medical records department, and a certain sum should be incorporated into their budget for retrieving records for audit. If records cannot be found, the management of the records department needs attention. Anyone who has worked in a hospital knows that running a records department is a nightmare. The staff always seem to be located in the basement, and they often have a miserable time trying to satisfy unreasonably disgruntled doctors. I believe that there needs to be a major investment in health records in this country.

I am sure that who does the coding and so on is a consultant-led responsibility. It is the job of a consultant to record the work that goes through his or her firm, unit or directorate. The division of purchasing from the provision of care is already ensuring better coding, because providers will not be paid unless they record their work.

Section 5

Achieving change

21 | The relationship between medical audit and the proposed performance procedures of the General Medical Council

Sir Robert Kilpatrick
President, General Medical Council

Earlier chapters have outlined how to change a harvest of 'good apples' into 'excellent apples'. Medical audit is a process of improvement and education. The proposed performance procedures of the General Medical Council (GMC), on the other hand, are intended to deal with bad apples, of which I do not believe there are many.

The General Medical Council

The purpose of the GMC and its role in relation to these audit activities are not well-known even amongst members of the medical profession. The following statement was made by a previous President at a lecture in Manchester in 1905:

> The Council is, in fact, neither a parliament for making professional laws nor a union for protecting professional interests. It may surprise some of you to learn that when the Council was created, ... the declared purpose of the Legislature was not to promote the welfare of professional men or professional corporations — it was not to 'put down quackery', or even to advance medical science. The object in view was simply the interest of the public.

The declared purpose of the legislature (which is of course Parliament, not the GMC) was simply the 'interest of the public'. Everything the Council does is on that basis, a basis given to the GMC by Parliament. This Act by Parliament in the United Kingdom, making a statutory provision for professional self-regulation, is very unusual worldwide.

The preamble of the initial Act in 1858 stated very clearly that:

> It is expedient that persons requiring medical aid should be enabled to distinguish qualified from unqualified practitioners.[1]

It has never been a function of the GMC to seek to eliminate the practice of medicine by unqualified persons. This is another striking feature of the law in the United Kingdom, which is very different from most other parts of the world, in particular Europe of which we are now an integral part. In this country medical treatment may be given by anyone, provided that the person does not pretend to have a medical qualification. Therefore, the preamble to the 1858 Act sets out the principle on which the Council was founded. The GMC still maintains a register of qualified individuals, but the word 'qualified' as used in 1858 has of course changed considerably in the intervening years.

The GMC has statutory jurisdiction in two principal areas in relation to doctors' fitness to practise. For a long time it had only one jurisdiction, namely that in relation to conduct. The jurisdiction applies in two areas:

- allegations of serious professional misconduct (which of course apply to most of the cases investigated by the Council); and
- criminal convictions.

In 1978, after publication of the Merrison Report on the GMC,[2] the health procedures were introduced to deal with doctors whose fitness to practise was seriously impaired by reason of a major health problem. The Council had previously dealt with such cases under its conduct procedures, which was obviously inappropriate. Thus, since 1978 the Council has had both conduct and health procedures.

Conduct procedures

I should like to describe further the conduct procedures, because they are inadequate in relation to cases arising from poor professional performance by doctors. The conduct procedures are formal, like criminal court proceedings, and are conducted in public, except for the Committee's *in camera* discussions in relation to its decisions. This is different from most professional self-regulation mechanisms, such as those which apply to solicitors, barristers, accountants, engineers and architects. It is only the 'medical' professional bodies, namely the GMC, the General Dental Council (GDC) and the United Kingdom Central Committee which conduct disciplinary proceedings in public.

The significant problem is that the conduct procedures have developed in a form very similar to criminal court procedures. The

Professional Conduct Committee is a *quasi* court of law (it is not a court of law, as it does not have the powers of a court), in that it uses the adversarial system of prosecution and defence, and all the evidence is given through the mouths of witnesses who are examined and cross-examined. Furthermore — and this is the crucial factor — the charge of serious professional misconduct brought against any doctor can only be in relation to specific facts. It is insufficient to make the allegation in general terms, for example, 'that Doctor Q's exhibition of professional care is poor'. This is the same as in the criminal courts, where the prosecution is not permitted to charge a person with being a bad citizen, but has to charge him or her with specific events and specific breaches of the law. The adversarial system is not appropriate for anything but specific events.

Thus, a difficulty or gap has been identified in the GMC's powers. Clearly, the Council has a problem in relation to investigating the cases of doctors when complaints or information are received indicating that the doctor's day-to-day, month-to-month, year-to-year pattern of professional care is deficient. The GMC does receive such complaints and information, including repeated complaints from different patients which cumulatively produce a picture of a deficient pattern of performance. For a long time this has been called 'incompetence'. However, the GMC is now reluctant to use this term, because 'competence' really describes what a doctor *can do,* whereas what really concerns the public and the GMC is what a doctor actually *does.*

The GMC has also recognised that its Professional Conduct Committee differs from a court of law. Unlike a jury, members of the Committee are allowed to question witnesses during a disciplinary inquiry, and of course also question the respondent doctor, if he goes on the witness stand. When that happens, and the Committee is, for example, investigating the doctor's treatment of a patient and looking at the record he has kept of that particular patient, the doctor's regular pattern of keeping records is commonly found to be deficient. For example, the doctor may tell the Committee that he never records a home visit or the prescriptions he issues. However, the Committee can pursue only the *specific* charges against the doctor.

Thus, the GMC has become acutely aware of deficiencies in its conduct procedures which prevent the investigation of cases of generally poor professional performance. In a small number of cases, adverse publicity concerning the Council's procedures has resulted.

Proposed performance procedures[3]

What action will be possible under the proposed performance procedures? First, they will investigate the doctor's pattern of professional care. The method of investigation will be to assess the doctor's standard of medical care by means of peer review, not by attempting to investigate specific events as in the conduct procedures. When deficiencies emerge in a doctor's performance, there is often no individual serious specific event which can be investigated. However, the accumulation of less serious events may add up to a pattern of seriously deficient performance.

Another major problem in relation to the conduct procedures is that the sanctions which the Professional Conduct Committee can apply to a doctor's registration generally mean that when the doctor returns to practice after suspension or after erasure and subsequent restoration, his or her standard of practice is inevitably worse, because he or she has been away from medical practice. Therefore, in the performance procedures, emphasis has been placed on dealing with poor performance by means of remedial, rehabilitative training.

It is sometimes suggested that the new performance procedures are intended by the GMC to deal with lesser, non-serious complaints. This is not the case. The gravity of the doctor's deficiency of performance would have to be comparable to the gravity of either serious professional misconduct or serious impairment of the doctor's fitness to practise as a result of ill health before the Council would institute proceedings against that doctor. The procedures will be developed in a way that will ensure equivalence and consistency in the assessment of a doctor's performance around the country. The Council would insist that the peer group conducting the assessment not only comprises two doctors from the same field of practice as the respondent doctor, but also one lay individual (this is now generally accepted by the profession). The GMC now has much experience with the contribution made by lay individuals on panels of the Professional Conduct and Health Committees. This is found to be invaluable, and the GMC would certainly wish to continue and extend it.

There will be, if enacted, three stages to the procedure, with an additional fourth stage (the Committee stage) in some cases:.

1. Preliminary screening of all complaints relating to performance.
2. Assessment of performance where there is evidence of serious deficiency.

3. Retraining where there appears to be significant deficiency in the doctor's performance, followed by a reassessment.
4. A new GMC Professional Performance Committee, which will deal with those doctors who refuse to co-operate with the procedures or whose performance remains seriously deficient, despite efforts at remedial training.

The above procedures are based on the health procedures. In developing them, it was realised that they could not follow the conduct procedures and be done adversarially. A person's health or poor performance cannot be assessed on the basis of investigation of specific events, but has to be assessed over a long period of time.

The screening mechanism for health, conduct and performance will be continued. All complaints, referrals and convictions are screened before a decision is made that the matter should go to a conduct panel, a health committee or (once these procedures have passed through Parliament) for assessment of the doctor's performance.

Screening is probably the most important part of the procedure. Of the 1,000 or so complaints from the public each year, on average only 50 doctors appear before the Professional Conduct Committee, and perhaps 25–30 are referred to the Health Committee. It seems likely that a similar number of doctors will be referred each year into the performance procedures. Many complaints are received which do not reach the level of gravity which would raise a doubt about the doctor's continued registration.

The GMC's only sanction is to restrict or remove the doctor's registration — a very serious matter. This is why the screening has to be to the level of 'serious misconduct', 'serious impairment' and, in future, 'serious deficiency of performance'. I cannot emphasise this enough. It is one of the areas where the GMC receives most criticism. Some lobbies say that the GMC ought to investigate every complaint. Those who wish to see the abolition of the GMC, the GDC, etc. suggest that an inspectorate be set up in place of all such authorities, which would inspect every complaint. However, many trivial complaints are received, related particularly to grief: the public believe that the measure of seriousness of a complaint relates to the *outcome* of the case, not to the doctor's *behaviour,* either in terms of deliberate misconduct or what would be called poor performance. However, the Council has to set aside the outcome and consider the degree to which the doctor's conduct or performance can be regarded as inappropriate. Many complaints (probably as large a section as any) are also received from the idiosyncratically mad.

After the screening stage, the new performance procedures will have an assessment stage, almost certainly locally. The GMC will now have to carry out a lot of research to ensure that the assessment procedure is valid, consistent and uniform. This will also apply to the proposed stage of rehabilitation and reassessment. Of course, it has to be accepted that there will inevitably be individuals who either will not take part in the procedure or are clearly irremediable. They will have to go finally to a Committee that can exert sanctions on registration.

Perfomance procedures and clinical audit

I suspect that the performance procedures will be on the statute-book by 1995. What will be their relationship to audit? The GMC has made it plain that it would not wish in any way to tie these procedures directly to medical audit; in other words, the GMC neither expects nor wishes to see direct referral of a case from the chairman of an audit committee, who clearly would be involved in the audit on a confidential basis. However, there will come a point with particular individuals when a health authority will feel that the individual should be referred to the GMC. (I suspect that there will be few such individuals because there is no question of a link between audit, which has to do with encouraging doctors, and the GMC procedures, which will be seen as a deterrent to poor practice). It is felt that such cases should be referred to the GMC by a responsible senior medical officer of the health authority. Serious cases are already referred under the conduct procedures, for example by regional directors of public health, and the same should probably apply when the performance procedures are in force. Such responsible officers would have to take the important decision to refer a case to the Council. They already have their own procedures in the National Health Service, but the GMC is the only authority which can affect all aspects of a doctor's practice. I know of one example of a doctor who, while suspended by one regional health authority, was employed by another. This is not unusual. The public interest has to be considered in relationship to a doctor's total registration.

Fitness to practise

One other important feature of the GMC's activities is in relation to fitness to practise. Guidance to the profession about professional standards is published by the GMC in a booklet sometimes

known as *The blue book.*[4] The questions may be asked, why does the
GMC not abandon self-regulation and have inspectors of doctors'
standards? In answer, I would point out that there are 140,000
practising doctors on the Register. We therefore have 140,000 doctors who can employ peer review, whether on a one-to-one basis,
within medical audit, or through a straightforward complaints
mechanism in the NHS. A significant proportion of the referrals
received each year come from individual doctors. If the complaint
is grave or serious, calling into question the doctor's continuing
registration, the matter can certainly be referred to the GMC.

References

1. *An Act to regulate the qualifications of practitioners in medicine and surgery.*
    2nd August 1858. (21 & 22 Vic. c.90)
2. Merrison AW (chmn). *Committee of enquiry into the regulation of the
    medical profession.* Report. Cmnd. 6018. London: HMSO, 1977
3. General Medical Council. Proposals for new performance
    procedures: a consultation paper. London: GMC, 1992
4. General Medical Council: *Professional conduct and discipline: Fitness to
    practice.* London: GMC, 1993

22 | How do we change systems of care in response to the findings of clinical audit?

Barbara Stocking

Chief Executive, Oxford Regional Health Authority; formerly Director, King's Fund Centre

Clinical audit is a cycle which moves through standard setting, to reviewing what the practice is against those standards, and then on to bringing about change. Many people are grappling with the question of how most effectively to bring about change. Understanding more about how change comes about would provide some insight into why clinical audit may or may not work in particular circumstances. What people have already tried to do to change clinical practice and the lessons learnt from these efforts both need to be considered.

The elements of change

It has first to be accepted that people are not entirely rational scientific beings. They do not automatically change to follow another practice that would be more effective. As Ogden Nash put it, 'I believe that people believe what they believe they believe'.

In thinking about change, it is necessary to consider three elements:

- the environment;
- the characteristics of the change itself; and
- the people involved in the change.

The environment

It may sometimes be impossible to bring about a change because either the national or the local environment for it is not right. An example of this occurred in some work I did some years ago on the introduction of regional secure units.[1] At first, the concept of such units was rejected, on the grounds that previously locked wards in

131

psychiatric hospitals had just been unlocked. Staff saw the establishment of secure units as a backwards step. Ten years later, the psychiatric hospitals were under threat of closure, as a result of new policies. Staff said then that these regional secure units were rather interesting, often being housed in brand-new buildings; and were seen as centres of excellence — the whole attitude changed. This is an example of something happening nationally that influences what could be done locally.

Characteristics of a change

Not all changes are the same. An analysis is needed of the characteristics of the particular change being attempted. Rogers summarised over 7,000 studies worldwide on bringing about change.[2] He considered all types of change, not just in health care, although change in clinical practice was included. The principles and characteristics of change can be seen to apply across a range of social systems.

First, if anybody is being asked to change, he or she will think about the *relative advantage* or *disadvantage* to him or herself. In the National Health Service (NHS), everybody likes to think that at the heart of everything they do they are primarily concerned about patients, and that whether or not change is accepted depends on the likely benefit of that change to patients. Of course, this is a central issue, but it is not the only aspect that people will consider when they think about advantages and disadvantages. They will think about routines, about convenience, and about their personal prestige and status. Change cannot be brought about without facing up to these realities.

Another significant feature is *compatibility*. Is an attempt being made to force somebody to change something that goes fundamentally against that person's beliefs and philosophies, all the concepts and practices taught in his or her professional training? If so, we will have a hard time. It does not mean to say that change is impossible, but it may take longer to bring about and may require different approaches.

The third characteristic is *complexity*, which is not always what it seems at face value. Complexity often means that many different people are involved. An example comes from research undertaken to bring about change in the time that patients are woken up in hospital.[1] It sounds simple: why cannot patients be woken up at 7.30 am instead of 6.30 am? However, what it means in reality is that night staff must negotiate with day staff about who is going to do what, the times at which the catering staff provide breakfast, the cleaners work and patients go to physiotherapy will all be different, and consultants may have to put up with the ward not being in order when they go round. Such a seemingly small change can have a dramatic degree of complexity.

The last two characteristics are not quite so critical. First, *observability*. People trying to bring about a change often take their team to look at something going on elsewhere. This can be quite strongly persuasive — unless the other place has many resources or really significant differences, in which case the team will then be convinced that they cannot do it back at home.

Finally, *triability*, trying it out. Is the change something that can be tried out for a short time? Although this makes change easier, trying out a new way of doing things often has the drawback that the change may not stick. If the new procedure is easy to try out, it is probably not necessary to have everybody's complete commitment. However, even if people formally accept a change, once the enthusiasts move away the change may slip away too. What is really at issue here is how to get change *built in* and carried on in the long-term.

The people involved in change

Different sorts of people take up change at different times.[1] This is common across social systems. The first people who adopt change are the *innovators*, the venturesome people. They are, however, seen as somewhat maverick, as not quite fitting into their social group. Sometimes what they do is good, and sometimes it may seem bizarre. The people who are influential in getting change in any system, however, are known as the *early adopters*. These are people whose key characteristic is that they are truly respected by their peers at national or at local level. Once they accept a change, the rest can be expected to follow. They are not necessarily (although they may be) the positional leaders, the key figures in named jobs. More *deliberate* and more *sceptical adopters* follow, and last come the *laggards*, those with traditional practices who will probably not change.

The process of bringing about change

With this knowledge of what happens in social systems, what have people done to try to bring about change in clinical practice? The immediate thought of most researchers and academic clinicians is that if only this information could get to the relevant people, they would undoubtedly respond. Information is necessary, but proves not to be sufficient. Publishing scientific papers and giving individual feedback to clinicians have been tried. The latter, however, does not seem to work well, probably because people are convinced that what they are already doing is right. If they are asked why they did not change when information was fed back, they say it is because they see themselves as outliers, with good reasons for their particular practices.

Researchers have also experimented with giving information and feedback in relation to particular standards or guidelines, having obtained some national or collegiate agreement to those standards (such as the guidelines of the Royal College of Radiologists).[3] Experience shows that more change is achieved using peer review processes in relation to guidelines when these concern diagnostic tests. There is more evidence of change in practice in relation to the ordering of investigations in radiology and pathology than in clinical treatment through these sorts of processes. For example, in relation to audit of one aspect of obstetric practice in Canada — high rates of Caesarean section — change did not occur even though virtually all the local obstetricians had acknowledged guidelines that should have reduced the rate substantially.[4] Guidelines were developed, with the involvement of the College of Obstetricians, including guidelines on trial of labour for women whose only indication for Caesarean section was one previous Caesarean section. The MacMaster group performed an experiment to explore how to get the change adopted. One arm used audit processes, but this was not successful in achieving change in rates of Caesarian section. The other arm of the experiment brought together opinion leaders, identified by the local obstetricians, informed them about the guidelines and gave some training about how they could persuade their colleagues to start changing practice. Some change locally was achieved by using this approach.

Education is always mentioned as a strategy to achieve change. Basic professional training has an enormous impact on people's beliefs and practices, but there is less evidence that people will change much afterwards, unless they are taught by respected and charismatic leaders in the field. Again, if people are not informed, they are not likely to change, but education alone may not be enough to bring about specific changes. There may also, of course, be a need for practical training, such as for laparoscopic surgery. We have not been very good in helping people acquire the skills to take on new procedures when this becomes necessary.

Financial incentives are another lever for change. It is known, particularly from the American and German systems of health care, that fee-for-service systems work in getting things done. This is not how health care system works in the UK, but even here there are examples showing that people will do things if they are paid for them — as has been seen recently with changes to the general practitioner contract. The problem is that financial incentives can be used to get people to do things for which there is no evidence of effectiveness, such as regular examinations of those aged over 75. This does not seem to be the way we really want to go: we want clinicians to reflect on their own practice and to make sure they always look at the evidence for what they are doing, and change their practice accordingly. Financial incentives *can* bring about change, but it is not possible to buy our way through all the improvements we are likely to want to make, nor do I see them as being beneficial in getting clinicians to look at their practice and to think about the evidence of effectiveness and efficiency.

The development of purchasing since the NHS reforms is another financial lever. An interesting question is how much purchasers will get into the business of changing clinical practice by specifying the standards they want and getting agreement to conform to practice guidelines. Purchasers are currently considering whether they should specify particular procedures and the standards they expect, or whether their approach will be to ask providers for assurance that they have their own quality procedures in place. Purchasers may, however, not only ask for systems of clinical audit to be in place, but also require particular issues to be audited, and to be informed of the results and of proposals for improvement.

People are important in the change process. The innovators and the early adopters, described in relation to Figure 1, tend to be those who go to national meetings and read medical journals. They may well be converted by the literature, but most people are converted by their colleagues. Patients can also be influential in changing practice, usually through the activities of associations of patients with particular disorders.

The media and patients together can change practice. One example comes from Switzerland, where there were high hysterectomy rates. In some cantons, but not others, the media published a lot of information about the appropriateness of hysterectomy. Doctors and other health professionals were aware of the media interest, but it was clear that there was patient pressure for a change in practice — which led to a reduction in rates of hysterectomy.[5]

Patients in the UK are not sufficiently well informed. If they are

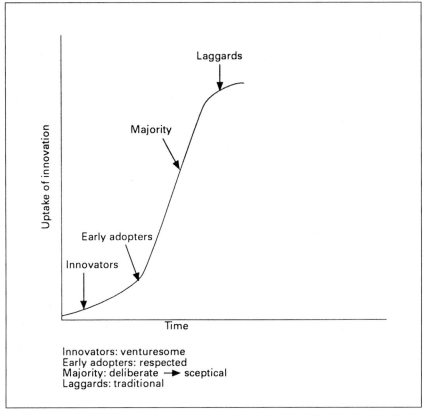

Fig 1. *Diffusion of uptake of innovations.* Reproduced with permission from Quality in Health Care[6]

to be agents to achieve changes in practice, they will need more information than it has been customary to give them.

Implications for audit

Whether or not audit *can* achieve a particular change needs to be assessed, and whether additional or alternative approaches are needed. People also need to be clear what they are trying to change. Do they all need to improve their practice, or in any particular instance is there one outlier who is really the problem? If it is the latter, the audit approach may not be the right way to deal with that individual, and his practice may have to be tackled more directly.

In the main, clinical audit has so far been concerned with local practice issues, although there are exceptions such as the National Confidential Enquiry into Perioperative Deaths.[7] This has resulted in changes in emergency surgery, and there are other changes in clinical practice that we would like to see on a national level. People accept change because they hear messages from a variety of sources, a variety of different people. If a new way of helping patients is reported in the *British Medical Journal* one week, a colleague talks to us about it the next, and the patients start discussing it with us the third week, we begin to wonder if there might be an issue. If a change is being promoted on a national level, we may need to operate on a variety of levels to bring about that change. All the relevant groups need to be targeted and brought to an understanding of change, an understanding that different people will respond to change in different ways, and that a variety of approaches may be needed. To achieve change may be difficult, but all of us should be aware of what has already been tried, what lessons have been learnt, and apply these lessons rather than keep on working in the dark.

References

1. Stocking B. *Initiative and inertia.* London: Nuffield Provincial Hospitals Trust, 1985: 95–138
2. Rogers B. *Diffusion of innovation,* 3rd ed. New York: Free Press, 1983
3. Fowkes FGR. *Strategies for change in the use of diagnostic radiology.* London: King's Fund, 1985 [project paper no. 57]
4. Lomas J, Enkin M, Anderson GM, *et al.* Opinion leaders *vs* audit and feedback to implement practice guidelines. *Journal of the American Medical Association* 1991; **265**: 2202–7
5. Domenighetti G, Luraschi P, Gutzwiller F, *et al.* Effect of information campaign by the mass media on hysterectomy rates *Lancet* 1988; **ii**: 140–3
6. Stocking B. Promoting change in clinical care. *Quality in Health Care* 1992; 1: 56–60
7. Campling EA, Devlin HB, Hoile RW, Lunn JN. *The report of the national Confidential Enquiry into Perioperative Deaths 1991/2.* London: NCEPOD Royal College of Surgeons 1993

DISCUSSION

Christopher Tallents: We have discussed changes in clinical practice in the public sector environment. Do you think changes in practice in the private sector environment will occur at the same rate? Is there as much pressure and motivation for change in that environment?

Barbara Stocking: Many health insurers are as anxious to achieve change as are purchasers in the NHS, and they have different incentives that might be used.

Anthony Hopkins: There are some contrary incentives operating in the private sector. For example, some health insurers also own hospitals. Their managers have a desire to keep their bed occupancy up and, at the same time, the insurers want to keep their costs per patient down.

In my experience, the standard of record keeping in most private clinics is not good. The tradition is that consultants working privately keep their notes in their consulting rooms and seldom, at least in London, make them available on the wards of private clinics.*

---

*Editor's note: Since the conference, the Royal College of Surgeons of England has set up a Private Practice Forum, with an audit sub-committee, to consider issues such as these.

Appendix A

Clinical audit in *HCHS: allocation of funds 1993/94

This Appendix is reproduced with permission from the text of an Executive Letter (EL (93) 34) from the NHS Management Executive.

---

1. We are pleased to inform you that £50.1M revenue has been centrally earmarked within the hospital and community health services budget for the continuing development of audit by health care professions in 1993/94. This sum comprises £41.9M for medical audit and £8.2M for audit of the nursing and therapy professions.

2. An additional allocation of £3.2M has also been made in order to facilitate and "pump prime" the development of multi-professional clinical audit.

3. Allocations to Regional Health Authorities and Special Health Authorities for 1993/94 are set out in Annex A to this letter. Payment will be made, upon receipt and approval of 1992/93 annual reports and 1993/94 forward plans, within twenty eight working days. Reports must be submitted by 31st July 1993. Details of the expected format and contents of the Medical Audit 1992/93 annual reports are attached (Annex C). Details regarding the format of nursing and therapy annual reports have already been circulated under separate cover. Reports should be sent to Elizabeth Kidd, Health Care Directorate, Room 3W37, Quarry House, Quarry Hill, Leeds LS2 7UE.

4. Funding for clinical audit from 1994/95 will be included in overall allocations to Regions. Regions will be expected to maintain and develop clinical audit and will be held accountable in this area; specific criteria on which performance will be measured after 1993/94 will be agreed at a later date.

The development of clinical audit

5. A policy statement setting out the main strands of the clinical audit strategy has been commissioned by the Department's

---

HCHS: Hospital and Community Health Services

Clinical Outcome Group (COG) and will be published shortly under separate cover.

6. In future years it is intended that a single audit programme will be in place, based on this policy, with a single annual report required. Structured reporting mechanisms are currently being developed in discussions with the professions for use during 1993/94.

7. To prepare for this change an additional sum of £3.2M has been made available to Regions for 1993/94 (See paragraph 2). These clinical audit development monies are set out in Annex A and will be issued with the main medical audit allocation.

8. In addition, during 1993/94, Regions are asked to promote the use of the clinical audit programme as part of the purchasers role in contracting. As an aid to discussion in this area a paper prepared by a working group of the Regional Medical Audit Co-ordinators Committee and Conference of Colleges Audit Group "Audit and the Purchaser/Provider Interaction" is attached at Annex B.

9. While the review of the Intermediate Tier function is taking place, it is essential that the development of clinical audit is sustained. The NHSME, therefore, needs to be assured that appropriate mechanisms and procedures are in place to under-pin that development. Regional General Managers are there-fore asked to set out their proposals for achieving this in a let-ter covering the 1992/93 annual report.

Prison Medical Service

10. Regions are asked to include arrangements to facilitate the development of audit within the Prison Medical Service within their overall plans for medical/clinical audit. Precise arrange-ments for funding those practices and units which will support prison doctors will be discussed with Regional Medical Audit Co-ordinators.

ANNEX A: Clinical audit in HCHS — allocation of Funds 1993/94

Region	Medical audit (1)	Nursing & therapy audit	Development of multi professional audit
	£000	£000	£000
Northern	2,128	438	218
Yorkshire	2,263	505	231
Trent	2,772	630	282
East Anglian	1,308	264	136
North West Thames	2,029	497	208
North East Thames	2,808	567	286
South East Thames	2,575	547	263
South West Thames	1,764	417	181
Wessex	1,526	389	158
Oxford	1,772	300	182
South Western	1,884	446	193
West Midlands	3,284	698	333
Mersey	1,540	336	159
North Western	2,819	569	287
SHAs–		80	
Hospital for Sick Children	139		14
National Hospital for Nervous Diseases	73		7
Moorfields Eye Hospital	68		7
Royal Marsden Hospital	90		9
Eastman Dental Hospital	47		5
National Heart & Chest	135		14
Bethlem Royal & Maudsley	106		11
Hammersmith & Queen Charlotte's	224		22
Total	*31,354*	*6,683*	*3,206*

(1) as 1992/93 allocation less £50,000 per Region "CESDI" monies. 1993/94 "CESDI" monies will be allocated by the Department's Health Promotion (Medical) Division. Regions have already been notified about their individual allocations in a letter to Regional General Managers dated 7 April 1993.

ANNEX B: Audit and the purchaser/provider interaction

Report of a Working Group of the Regional Medical Audit Coordinators' Committee and Conference of Colleges' Audit Working Group members (February 1993)

Introduction

There is widespread debate about the future of audit in the context of the purchaser/provider interaction and contracting for services. This requires guidance, not least because ring-fenced funding for audit (medical, nursing and paramedical) will cease. However, the distribution and management of funds is a means to an end. The ultimate goal of audit is to improve the quality of care provided to patients: it is with this shared goal in mind that this paper has been written. It draws upon the experiences and discussions still ongoing in two regions, including a survey of purchaser views across several regions.

Principles and vision

Before developing guidance, it is necessary to make explicit the principles and vision upon which the guidance depends. Within five years, it is to be hoped that:

- Audit will be largely multidisciplinary (clinical) audit and part of hospital-wide quality management programmes;
- Audit will be informed by purchaser/provider and public/patient as well as professional (college) priorities;
- The findings of audit will inform service development and purchasing;
- Audit will be an integrated part of routine activity and continuing professional education;
- Audit will increasingly demonstrate its effectiveness and cost effectiveness to provider, purchaser and the public;
- Audit will increasingly focus upon outcomes and their relationships to the processes of care;
- Audit will be a shared process bridging primary and secondary care sectors.

In order for audit to develop within the principles and vision described, a number of actions will need to occur. These include recognition by purchasers and providers, and by management and clinicians, of different perspectives within the overriding principles and purpose of audit.

Clinician/management interface at provider level

Before the purchaser/provider interface can be developed, it is equally important to clarify the management–clinician interface at provider level.

In many provider units management will be exercised at specialty level by clinical directors. Whilst audit remains a clinically led quality improvement process, it is clear that non-clinical input and support is crucial to the development of effective audit programmes, both from those directly involved (e.g. audit assistants) and those indirectly involved (e.g. unit general management).

Clinicians will find it easier to develop supported and resourced audit programmes if managers and clinical directors are:

a) well informed about the methods, function, value and general results of audit;
b) convinced that audit is of benefit to patients, the unit and its staff;
c) assured that effective audit leading to quality improvement is taking place;
d) able to create a culture that supports and stimulates the development of audit and other quality improvement programmes.

There is a clear need to improve and understand the management/clinician interface at unit level. The role of unit management in the development of audit is thus to:

1. understand the purpose, role and function of audit;
2. understand audit as part of the unit based quality improvement programme or strategy;
3. understand the resource and support needs for audit, particularly the role of an audit office, audit assistants/facilitators, and the information needs of audit;
4. ensure that the information and IT needs of audit are integrated into wider unit based information and IT strategies (including resource management and HISS);
5. ensure that the recurring cost of audit programmes are built into contract pricing once ring-fenced monies cease;
6. ensure that the contracts negotiated for services and the purchaser-provider interface on audit are managed appropriately;
7. respond to the resource implications of the findings of audit;
8   receive and, where appropriate, act upon the findings of audit;
9. most importantly, support and stimulate a culture of continuous quality improvement across the unit.

In order for this to occur, the unit audit leads/chairmen and audit committee have a responsibility to:

1. ensure open discussion about the resource needs for audit and the resource implications of the findings of audit;
2. provide unit management with the general results of audit, in particular demonstrating change and quality improvement as a result of the audit programme;
3. ensure appropriate budgetary management;
4. contribute to contract negotiation discussions with major purchasers of services with particular reference to the quality elements of contracts;
5. include appropriate management input/representation on the audit committee;
6. ensure, in discussion with unit management, that audit programmes are consistent with the priorities of both clinicians and the goals of the organisation within which they work.

Through these mechanism the provider unit should develop a corporate view of audit, central to the organisation's function.

The purchaser/provider interface

The different perspectives of purchasers and providers with reference to quality are perhaps best summarised as:

- Purchasers are concerned with contracting for the right services, and assuring themselves that providers have effective quality improvement mechanisms;
- Providers are concerned with doing what they do well, and having mechanisms for continually improving what they do;
- Both have a joint role to play in contract negotiation and specification, and continuing dialogue on services purchased or provided, including significant clinical input into the contract negotiation process.

Purchasers have a legitimate interest in being assured that effective audit is under way and in receiving the general results of audit to enable such a judgement to be made. They will also have views on subjects or topics that audit and quality improvement programmes should address at provider level. Such views will be informed, for instance, by surveys of patient or GP opinion. Audit topics should be negotiated and agreed bi-laterally between purchaser and provider clinical audit leads. There will be some data requirements negotiated between purchaser and provider that may best be obtained and collated through the audit programme. However, it is clearly important that the audit programme is not stifled by inappropriate demands from purchasers and that purchasers, through the contract negotation process, agree to meet the resource needs of audit.

The purchaser provider interaction on audit will be best managed if:

a   purchasing organisations understand the purpose, role, function and limitations of audit;
b   provider based clinicians have a key role in discussions with purchasers on audit and contract negotiation.

Guidance for Regions

In order to meet the above, Regions should ensure that:

- At Unit level, managers and clinicians are jointly involved in the development, resourcing and assessment of audit programmes;
- Purchasers and providers should develop a mechanism for open discussion, at least annually, between themselves on audit priorities, progress and outcomes;
- Directors of Public Health and their departments at district level should take an enhanced role in audit and quality improvement from the purchaser perspective. Membership on audit committees should be encouraged (both MAAGs and LMACs);
- LMACs should include unit management and primary care representation;
- Providers should set up a multidisciplinary quality group or committee, in addition to or in place of LMACs;

- Clinicians and managers should ensure that there is strong clinical input into contract discussions and quality specifications;
- Purchasers and providers should ensure that all contracts make appropriate reference to audit;
- Audit committee chairmen should present their annual reports to their local DHA(s)/FHSA(s);
- DHAs and FHSAs should discuss audit annually and ensure that purchasing decisions are informed by the results of audit.
- Regions should support or facilitate workshops to enable discussion on audit between purchaser and provider teams, in order to develop action plans for progress;
- There should be an agreed format for the flow of audit information and progress reports/annual forward programmes from hospital and community health services to districts and GP fund holders.
- Providers of IHSM and similar courses for health service management should include audit and quality improvement as part of the course.

Conclusions

At present audit largely by-passes the purchaser-provider interaction. Increasingly, it will need to become, on the one hand, integrated into provider based quality improvement programmes and, on the other hand, developed in the context of the purchaser-provider split and contracting.

This guidance should enhance the development of audit within the context of the NHS reforms.

References

Cook GA. *Purchasers' Views on the Medical Audit Programme: A telephone survey of views.* North Western Regional Health Authority 1992.

Harman D and Martin G. *Medical Audit and the Manager: A discussion document.* Health Services Management Centre, Birmingham 1991.

Paper prepared by:
Richard Thomson, Senior Lecturer in Public Health Medicine, Department of Epidemiology & Public Health, University of Newcastle upon Tyne.
Gary Cook, Regional Audit Co-ordinator, North Western Regional Health Authority
Paul Lelliott, Consultant Psychiatrist, The Royal College of Psychiatrists.
Ian Baker, Consultant in Public Health Medicine, Bristol & District Health Authority.
Ray Godwin, Audit Chairman, Royal College of Radiologists, Faculty of Clinical Radiology, West Suffolk Hospital.

ANNEX C: Format of medical audit reports 1992/93

Annual reports should cover the following categories:

    1. Financial report
    2. Progress with forward plan
    3. Audit activity
    4. Audit support staff
    5. Regional initiatives
    6. Forward plan 1993/94

Five copies of the report including one unbound copy should be sent as soon as possible, but no later than 31 July 1994 to Elizabeth Kidd, Health Care Directorate, Room 3W37, Quarry House, Quarry Hill, Leeds LS2 7UE.

1. Financial information

Financial Reports should include details of expenditure under the following headings.

Receipts
Revenue   Carried forward
            DH top-sliced allocation: HCHS Medical Audit
                                          CESDI
            Other (e.g. primary care audit funds)

Capital   Carried forward
            Converted from Revenue

Deployment
Revenue   District allocations
            Regional audit office
            Training & education
            1–3 Year regionally managed projects
            Ongoing projects (eg CESDI)
            Public Health support

Capital   Nature of purchase and location/project

2. Progress with 92/93 forward plan

Regional Health Authorities directed their 92/93 forward plan towards achieving the following objectives:

●   demonstrating that Medical Audit is leading to improvement in quality of care and health outcome;

- securing acceptance of Medical Audit as a routine element of patient care;
- making Medical Audit an integral part of postgraduate and continuing education in all specialties;
- achieving change through a process of setting standards and comparing practice with them;
- using the generalised results of national and local audits to inform the provision of healthcare for populations.

The report should reflect progress with all of these objectives, in particular including examples of good medical audits which have changed medical practice and led to improvements in the quality of health care.

3. Audit activity

The report should attempt to quantify audit activity by District/Trust and specialty along the following lines:

Frequency of Audit meetings

Proportion of doctors participating

Number and/or proportion of Audits which were:–
Multiprofessional
Across the primary/secondary interface

Number and/or proportion of Audits resulting in:–
Change in practice
Setting standards
Guidelines

Number and/or proportion of re-auditted topics

It is acknowledged that this quantitative data does not necessarily reflect the quality of audit. Structured reporting mechanisms are currently being developed with the professions and should be available during 1993/94.

4. Audit support staff

There is a relationship between the level of audit activity and the degree of support provided by audit support staff. Details should therefore be included on the level and type of audit support infrastructures in place at District or Trust level.

Details of the support staff establishment should include:

Number of WTE (Whole Time Equivalents)
Grade
Job Title/description
Contract type (permanent/temporary)

5. Regional initiatives

The Annual Report should contain details of all Regional initiatives including:

Training and education programmes
Regionally funded audit projects
Specialty Audit Groups/Regional Audits

6. Forward plan 1993/94

The forward plan should include developments of audit directed to the objectives outlined in section 2 with particular regard to the development of patient centred multi-professional audit and audit across the primary/secondary interface.